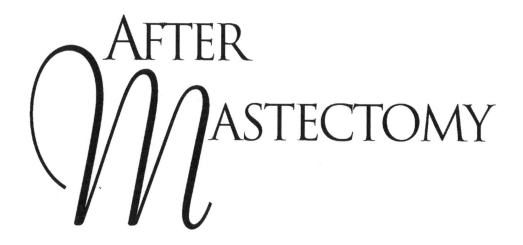

AFTER MASTECTOMY

HEALING PHYSICALLY *and* EMOTIONALLY

ROSALIND BENEDET, R.N.

Addicus Books
Omaha, Nebraska

An Addicus Nonfiction Book

Copyright 2003 by Rosalind Benedet. All rights reserved. No part of this publication may be reproduced, stored in a retrieval system, or transmitted in any form or by any means, electronic, mechanical, photocopied, recorded, or otherwise, without the prior written permission of the publisher. For information, write Addicus Books, Inc., P.O. Box 45327, Omaha, Nebraska 68145.

ISBN# 1-886039-61-5

Cover design by Peri Paloni
Illustrations by Bob Hogenmiller and Jack Kusler
Typesetting by Linda Dageforde

This book is not intended to be a substitute for a physician, nor does the author intend to give medical advice contrary to that of an attending physician's.

Library of Congress Cataloging-in-Publication Data

Benedet, Rosalind Dolores.
    After mastectomy : healing physically and emotionally / Rosalind
Benedet.
        p. ; cm.
Includes index.
    ISBN 1-886039-61-5 (alk. paper)
1. Mastectomy—Popular works.
    [DNLM: 1. Mastectomy—rehabilitation—Popular Works. 2. Breast
Neoplasms—therapy—Popular Works. WP 910 B462a 2003] I. Title.

RD667.5.B46 2003
618.1'9059—dc21   2003002584

Addicus Books, Inc.
P.O. Box 45327
Omaha, Nebraska 68145
Web site: www.AddicusBooks.com

Printed in the United States of America
10 9 8 7 6 5 4 3 2 1

Contents

Acknowledgments

I would like to thank my patients for helping make this book possible. Were it not for what they have taught me, I could not have written this book. Their strength and resilience have inspired me. Their wisdom has enriched my life.

I would also like to thank Loren Eskenazi, M.D., who has been a role model to me. She is a skilled healer who helps women use the experience of cancer and surgery as a "transformative experience." I also thank her for permission to reprint photos from her book *Reconstructing Aphrodite*, a testimony to her work and to the internal and external beauty of women.

In the middle of difficulty lies opportunity.

—Albert Einstein

Introduction

I am an oncology nurse. In our hospital, I'm the one who meets with a woman and tells her the results of her biopsy. I'm the person that tells her that she has breast cancer. It is not an easy message to deliver. And, more importantly, it's not an easy message for women to absorb. Most women are understandably stunned. It's hard for them to believe they have breast cancer, particularly since most women feel fine at the time of diagnosis.

In my work, I help women thought their journey, from diagnoses to follow-up care. In my twelve years as an oncology nurse, I have learned many things along the way. My patients have been my best teachers. They have shown me that physical and emotional recovery is a process that requires time, effort, information, and open communication. My patients have also taught me that the diagnosis of cancer can be used as a powerful motivator for a healthier life physically and emotionally.

It is my hope that, through this book, I may pass on some of the many lessons these women have taught me. Lessons to help you in both your physical and emotional recovery.

1

Recovering after Surgery

Even though a mastectomy is major surgery, most women are surprised that they feel much better than they expected they would by the time they return home. Still, you'll need to take it easy for awhile. You may have the help of friends and relatives, but you'll probably find that most of your care will be up to you. This chapter is to help you during the first few days that you're home.

Energy and Bed Rest

Although you probably won't have a great deal of post-surgical discomfort by the time you arrive home, you will probably feel fatigued both from the surgery and from the medications you received. In fact, your first impulse may be to go to bed and stay there until you feel more energetic. But bed rest is not encouraged, because inactivity leads to more fatigue.

How much can you do and how soon? Follow the guidelines from your doctor but a good rule of thumb is to "do what you feel capable of doing."

Generally, you can resume your normal, daily activities such as grooming, bathing, dressing, and eating, without assistance.

However, for more strenuous household tasks, you will need the help of family and friends. Avoid any heavy lifting, pushing, or pulling for six weeks. But you may do light household activities such as washing a few dishes, making a simple meal, and setting the table. Be gentle in using your affected arm. There's a natural tendency to favor the side where the operation was done and to hold your arm stiffly at your side. Try to keep your affected arm, neck, and shoulder relaxed.

Managing Pain

You will be more likely to experience some post-surgical pain if your operation involved the removal of lymph nodes. If you do feel some discomfort, there are a number of steps you can take to ease the pain.

Prescription Pain Medication

If your doctor has given you a prescription for a pain medication, be sure to have the prescription filled right away, and take the prescribed dose as recommended. Some women resist taking these medications because they worry about dependency. But in all likelihood, you won't need to take a prescription painkiller for more than a few days and nights, so dependency is not really an issue.

Take your pain medication before pain intensifies. If you wait until the pain starts, you'll have to endure the discomfort while you are waiting for the medication to work. And you will probably take more medication in the long run.

Over-the-Counter Medications

Side effects of prescription drugs, especially sleepiness and constipation, bother some women. These side effects are rarely if ever a problem with over-the-counter (OTC) pain relievers such as Tylenol. If you begin taking an OTC pain reliever along with your prescription medication on a regular schedule, you should be able to cut back on the prescribed pain medication. Keep your doctor informed about what medications you are taking. And be sure to avoid OTC products that contain aspirin or other medications such as Advil, Anacin, Motrin, and Aleve. These medicines have a "blood thinning" effect that promotes bleeding.

Cold Packs and Heat Packs

If you had lymph nodes removed, your greatest discomfort is usually in the underarm area. Cold packs, and later warm packs, may help relieve the discomfort. An ice treatment is best right after surgery.

You can purchase soft gel packs (the kind athletes use) at a pharmacy and keep them in the freezer until you're ready to use them. A bag of frozen peas or frozen cranberries works just as well. Wrap the cold bag in a soft cotton towel so that it doesn't come into direct contact with your skin. If this treatment helps, you can leave the ice pack in place for as long as twenty minutes. Then, remove the pack for ten minutes before applying it again.

Heat may be comforting, but you must wait at least seven days after surgery before using a heating pad, because it can increase post-surgery swelling. The area around your incision will be numb, so be careful not to burn yourself with a heating pad. Use only a low to moderate heat setting.

Caring for Your Dressing

You'll have a dressing that needs to stay in place for five days, or until your follow-up visit with your surgeon. You may have a simple gauze dressing, a bulky gauze dressing, or an elastic dressing that covers your entire torso.

Keeping the dressing dry is essential. If the dressing becomes wet, the incision won't heal properly, and the risk of infection increases. You may sit in a shallow bath as soon as you wish, but postpone taking a shower. You may need help bathing; or you might choose to take a sponge bath.

Caring for Your Drain

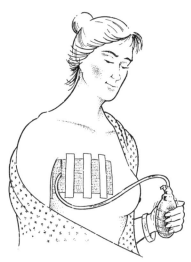

You'll be instructed how to empty your drain, which will collect blood and fluids that normally collect at the incision site.

You will likely have a "drain," just under the skin to remove blood and fluids that collect during the healing process. Your hospital nurse will review the instructions with you before you leave the hospital. Each day, the amount of drainage should decrease. The color of the fluid will change over the days, from red to light pink.

If you notice there is no drainage, you may have a blocked drain. The following "milking" technique may open it. Pinch off the end of the drain nearest your body with your left hand and run wet gauze a short distance down the tube with the right hand. While still holding the tube with the right hand, release the left, move it down behind the right hand, and pinch the tube again. Resume the milking action with your right hand, pinching off with your left hand each time so the suction action pulls any blockage down the tube. If this technique doesn't work, and you're still not getting drainage, call your surgeon.

If you notice that your drainage is increasing rather than decreasing, you are probably overdoing it—overusing your affected arm. Use that arm more gently, and notice if there is less drainage the next day. If the drainage continues to increase, call your surgeon.

Meals at Home

Keeping good nutrition in mind, you may eat foods that appeal to you when you first arrive home. It's important to drink plenty of water and other hydrating liquids—they help the body's cells do their work. Non-caffeinated drinks are recommended because caffeine is actually dehydrating. Chapter 3 offers more information on healthful nutrition.

Managing Constipation

Constipation may result from general anesthesia and pain medications. Here are some specific recommendations to help with constipation:

- Drink 10 glasses of hydrating liquids a day.
- Try drinking a cup of coffee or tea in the morning.
- Increase the fiber in your diet with fruits, vegetables, and bran cereal.
- As you resume exercise, pay special attention to walking, which stimulates the movement in your colon that brings on a bowel movement.

- Eat at least five prunes a day or drink a daily glass of prune juice. Prunes have a nutritional component that gives them a well-deserved reputation for promoting bowel movements.

Sleeping at Night

Sleeping well is essential for physical and emotional stamina. However, you may find falling asleep a challenge in the weeks after surgery. You will likely be more comfortable if you position several pillows around yourself. The pillows also help minimize post-surgical swelling. Place several large pillows behind your back, so that your body is at a forty-five degree angle. Use more pillows to raise the arm on your affected side (or on both sides). Your arms should be higher than your heart when you're leaning back comfortably against the pillows.

The following guidelines will also help you get the best rest possible:

- Keep your bedroom dark, quiet, and cool. The atmosphere of your bedroom should be calm and relaxing. If you have a computer or piles of paperwork on the desk in your bedroom, move the desk to another room.
- Establish a sleep routine. Go to bed at the same time every night. Set your alarm clock so that you wake up the same time each morning, then get up with the alarm—even if you are tired. If you need a nap later in the day, make sure that you set the alarm again, for just one hour. Napping longer than that is likely to interfere with your night's sleep.

- Establish a pleasurable and relaxing sleep ritual. If you are taking pain medication, take a pill forty-five minutes before you go to bed. Each night before you fall asleep, listen to soothing music, read a relaxing book, or say prayers.
- Avoid turning on bright lights. Leave a night light on in case you wake up during the night and need to find your way to the bathroom. To help yourself fall asleep again, repeat your relaxing sleep ritual.
- Eat a "sleep-promoting" snack. Foods that contain the amino acid tryptophan help promote sleep, but you need to eat them at least an hour before you go to bed. These foods include cottage cheese, yogurt, turkey, fish, and bananas.
- Avoid "wake-up" foods that may cause indigestion. These include spicy foods, alcohol, citrus juice, and beverages that are carbonated or caffeinated, chocolate, peppermint, fatty or greasy foods, and whole milk dairy products.
- Avoid drinking within four hours of your bedtime. (To avoid going to the bathroom.)
- If you are experiencing sleep problems because of depression, stress, and anxiety, try writing down your concerns in a journal or jotting down questions that you need to ask your doctors.

Finally, if you are following these recommendations and still having trouble with sleeplessness, speak to your doctor. He or she may be able to prescribe a medication that can help you sleep. Remember, sleeping well is essential to your recovery.

Managing Hot Flashes

If you experience hot flashes, you can take a number of steps that may reduce their frequency or intensity. Here are a few suggestions:

- Dress in layers. If you wear a sleeveless shirt under a sweater or jacket, you can quickly remove the outer layer and immediately feel more comfortable. Avoid turtleneck shirts or sweaters.
- Avoid certain foods that are known to trigger hot flashes, such as caffeine, alcohol and spicy foods.
- Avoid hot tubs, saunas, hot baths, and hot showers.
- In hot weather, try to stay in an air-conditioned area where you can get some relief if a hot flash comes on.
- Sleep in a cold room at night, under light covers, in a light, sleeveless nightgown and no socks.
- Stay well hydrated.
- Take a daily thirty-minute walk.

Your First Post-Operative Visit

At your first follow-up visit to the surgeon, usually five days after surgery, your doctor will remove your dressing and check your incision. If you have had a drain or drains in place, they could be taken out at this time.

Surgeons use different kinds of stitches, and some of them don't have to be removed at all. Absorbable stitches, as the name implies, dissolve on their own. The steri-strips (a special kind of tape) that are placed over absorbable stitches usually remain in place for about seven to ten days, so your surgeon won't remove them during this visit. The strips will fall off on their own.

If your pathology report is ready, your surgeon will review the results with you. Your surgeon will also go over the status of your lymph nodes, if they were sampled.

Looking at Your Incision

Your first post-operative visit may be the first time you're able to look at your incision. Many women find that it's difficult to do. Some women prefer to have a partner or friend with them when the surgeon removes the bandages. Initially, if you are having difficulty looking at yourself in the mirror, try looking down at your incision. Gradually you'll become more comfortable looking in the mirror.

Early on, your arm, underarm, and chest will be swollen from the surgery. Post-operative swelling is temporary, and it's a normal part of healing. After about six weeks, the swelling lessens. In the meantime, you can minimize swelling by following these guidelines:

- Don't overuse your arm. Gentle, normal movements are fine, but this is no time to be lifting boxes or spending a lot of time at the keyboard.
- When sitting or lying, rest your arm comfortably on several pillows so that your hand and forearm are higher than your heart.
- Perform the "Arm Pumps," described in Chapter 2 at least three times a day.

You may also notice bruising in the chest and underarm area. This, too, is normal, but will disappear in about six weeks. The bruise marks will gradually change colors, from a dark blue to purple to a light yellow.

Caring for Your Incision

Although it may be difficult, it is important to look at your incision daily for signs of infection: increased redness, swelling, warmth, pain around the incision, or drainage. If you notice staining that is increasing in size on your underclothes, call the surgeon's office immediately. Tell the medical staff the size as well as the color of the drainage. A red stain indicates bleeding; a greenish stain indicates infection. Normal drainage is yellowish pink or brown.

You are encouraged to wash your incision with mild soap and water to help reduce the risk of infection. Don't be afraid to touch it. Since the area will be numb, it may feel unusual. Use the pads of your fingers and make circular motions, working your way from one end of the incision to the other. You can use a washcloth if you prefer, but no harsh scrubbing.

After you wash, pat the area until it's completely dry, always using a fresh, clean towel to reduce the risk of infection. Some surgeons prescribe a topical antibiotic ointment to be gently applied to the incision after bathing.

Don't submerge your torso in water until your surgeon gives you the okay. Once the drain or drains have been removed, you will also have the option of taking a shower the next morning. Shower with your back to the shower head, avoiding the full force of the water on your incision.

The Scar

As your incision heals, a scar will form; it will be dark pink at first, but will fade to light pink. Over time (sometimes as long as a year), the scar will fade and take on the color of your skin. When you run your finger over the scar, you will feel a firm ridge, called a "healing ridge," that softens as healing progresses.

While the scar is healing, it may itch. You can help relieve the itching by massaging a mild, unscented lotion into the skin.

Possible Complications

Although an infection at the site of the incision is unlikely, be alert to signs of infection, mentioned earlier.

Sometimes a pocket of fluid, called a *seroma*, develops in the armpit. If this occurs, you will feel the bulge when you rub your arm against your body. A seroma may feel uncomfortably large. While it usually shrinks by itself in about six weeks, you and your surgeon may decide that you will be more comfortable if it's drained.

The quick procedure is done in the doctor's office. A very small needle is inserted into the seroma, and the fluid is removed. There is little if any pain during the procedure.

Noting Sensory Changes

As you touch your incision, chest, and underarm, you will discover that some areas lack sensation and others are extremely sensitive to touch. Over the next eighteen months, you will probably experience ever-changing sensations. You may feel sharp pain or a dull aching, heaviness, stiffness, or burning in your chest, arm, shoulder blade or rib cage on the side of your surgery. These sensations may increase when you're tired or feeling stressed. Changes in the weather can also make a difference.

The actual incision site will probably remain numb permanently since the nerve supply was cut. You may have some slight tingling sensations, but these will dissipate over time.

If lymph nodes were removed, additional nerves may have been severed or stretched. As a result, you may feel some numbness in your armpit and on the back of your arm. You may regain some feeling in these areas.

At times you may also feel as if you still have the breast that was removed. This "phantom breast" experience is common. Some women find it disturbing, while others are comforted by it. Over time, the sensation lessens.

Driving

You can begin driving again when you feel ready, as long as you are no longer taking narcotic pain medication. If the cross-strap of your seatbelt is uncomfortable, slip a small pillow between the belt and your chest.

At first, it may feel uncomfortable to turn the wheel, especially when you're parallel parking. However, such movement will not harm or reopen your incision.

Going Back to Work

Your readiness to return to work needs to be weighed against your progress in healing. Is your job physically or emotionally demanding? Discuss your working conditions with your surgeon. Of course, any further treatment you may require may influence your return to work.

Once you are back at work, should you tell your co-workers that you have had a mastectomy? Some women prefer to keep the matter private. On the other hand, if no one knows, they can't offer the support they may otherwise offer. You need to do what feels right for you. If you join a support group where some members have already gone back to work, you can learn from some of their experiences.

As for legal rights, under the Federal Rehabilitation Act of 1973, federal employers or companies receiving federal funding cannot discriminate against cancer survivors. But state laws vary, and federal legislation doesn't affect the private sector.

2

Your Exercise Program

Often, when we think of recuperating from surgery, we think of getting cozy in bed, eating treats, and watching television. Granted, those activities may play a part in your recovery, but the sooner you begin moving and exercising, the sooner your body will recover. In fact, if you feel like it, take a short walk your first day home from the hospital.

On your second day home from the hospital, you may begin doing gentle stretching of the muscles in the arms, neck, shoulder, and chest. Then, in about three weeks, you may begin doing some light weight lifting exercises. Of course, it is important to start slowly. You can gradually increase the pace and intensity of exercising.

Importance of Stretching

Regular stretching is essential for achieving flexibility. The stretch will feel uncomfortable but should not be unbearable. Scar tissue is inelastic, and you're pulling on it when you stretch, which explains the discomfort. But that pulling sensation is an indication that you are making progress. As you continue to stretch every day, you will gradually regain your flexibility and begin to feel more comfortable. Don't worry. You won't open up your incision.

The following guidelines apply to all stretching exercises.

- Stretch once or twice a day, starting the second day that you're home from the hospital.
- Each time you stretch, try to reach a little bit farther than you did before. Stop and hold the stretch as soon as you feel your incision pulling.
- Hold the stretch for at least fifteen seconds. Do not bounce when stretching.
- Remember to breathe before, during, and after each stretch.

Before You Begin Stretching

Get Comfortable

When you're doing arm stretches or other forms of exercise indoors, keep the room quiet and dimly lit. The room temperature should be moderate. If you're doing floor exercises, it's advisable to have a carpet, rug, or exercise mat.

Before you exercise, make sure you feel steady and confident, that you can keep your balance. At first, you may want to sit on the edge of the bed or on a comfortable chair with both feet touching the floor. Take three deep breaths, then begin.

The best clothing is loose and comfortable such as sweat pants with an elastic waistband. Always remove your shoes.

Get Relaxed

It's helpful to do relaxation exercises before and after exercise. When you are completely relaxed, your respiration slows, your blood pressure falls, and the rate of your heartbeat decreases. One way to relax is through the use of *extended exhalations.* To do these, lie down or sit in a comfortable chair. Close your eyes and focus all your attention on your breathing. Inhale and exhale slowly and deeply for at least three long breaths. Inhale through your nose. Exhale through your mouth.

Continue focusing on your breathing, making your exhalations longer than your inhalations. Then try closing your mouth and exhaling through your nose. Maintaining the slow, steady, deep rhythm of breathing, continue to inhale and exhale.

As you settle into a steady breathing pattern, you may find that your mind wanders. If so, shift your focus back to your breath. Some women like to think of healing words, focusing on a word or phrase like " hope," "love," or "healing energy."

Shoulder Shrugs

You may notice that your neck, shoulder, and arm feel tight, stiff, and sore on the side of your surgery. For relief, try several shoulder shrugs.

To keep your shoulders flexible, you may begin this simple stretch the day after you return home. Since your arms remain at your sides, this stretch can be done easily even if you have a drain. Do shoulder shrugs at least once every day, or before you begin doing other stretches and exercises.

Position: Stand with your arms by your side.

Motion: Raise your shoulders up towards your ears, hold for a few seconds, and then lower them.

Repetitions: 3

Arm Stretching Exercises

Arm Pumps

After surgery you may notice that your upper arm is swollen. Anytime you notice swelling in your hand or arm, it indicates a build-up of lymphatic fluid. Arm pumps increase lymphatic drainage, reducing the swelling.

Start the arm pump exercise the day after surgery. Arm pumps can be done even while the drains are still in place. Repeat the exercise at least once every day—or any time you notice swelling in your hand or arm.

(But be sure to let your surgeon know about the swelling.)

Position: Seated, with your affected arm resting on pillows, so it's positioned higher than your heart. (For increased comfort, you might also want a pillow supporting the small of your back.)

Motion: While making a fist, bring your hand toward your shoulder. Make a hard fist, squeezing hard and holding it for a few seconds. Then make a hard muscle your biceps. Lower your arm again, relaxing and opening your hand.

Repetitions: 5

This is a good exercise to use on an airplane the decreased atmospheric pressure can causes swelling, especially since you can do it while seated.

Arm Raises

Doing arm raises will also keep your shoulders flexible. You may begin this stretch in the first week, but if the drains are still in, be sure you never lift your arms higher than your shoulders.

Position: Stand with your arms by your side and your shoulders relaxed.

Motion: Keeping your arms straight, slowly raise both arms in front of you until your hands are level with your shoulders, palms

facing the floor. Then, slowly, separate your arms until they're outstretched at your sides. Finally, lower your arms to your sides.

Repetitions: 5

Climbing

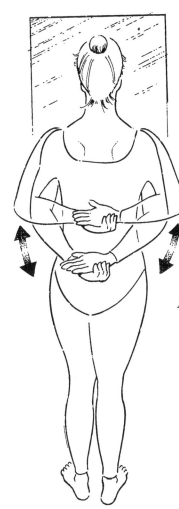

You may begin this exercise two to six weeks after your mastectomy, after your drain is removed. You'll increase the flexibility in the muscles of your affected arm as you reach for the middle of your back.

Position: Stand straight.

Motion: Place your hands behind your lower back and clasp them together. Slowly slide your clasped hands up the center of your back. Stop when you start to feel your incision pulling. Hold that position for 15 seconds.

Repetitions: 1

Clasp-Lift Stretch

This stretch helps to increase the range of motion of your affected arm. Since you'll have to move your arms above shoulder level, don't attempt this until your drains are removed. Even if you did not have a drain, you should wait until the second week after surgery before you try this stretch.

Position: Stand upright.

Motion: Clasp your hands together in front of you. Slowly raise your hands toward the ceiling. Make sure your elbows are not bent, and your arms are straight. Stop when you feel your incision pulling. Hold that position for 15 seconds.

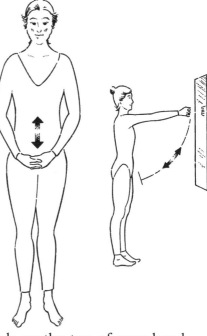

With your fingers still clasped, bend your arms and rest your clasped hands on the top of your head. Gradually extend your elbows back. Hold for 15 seconds. Keep your head upright.

Do this stretch daily. Each day that you repeat this exercise, you will find that you can move your clasped hands farther towards the back of your head. With each repetition, continue to challenge yourself by sliding your clasped hands a little farther over your head. The first time you do the "Clasp-Lift Stretch," you may only be able to touch the upper part of your forehead. Over time, you will eventually be able to move your clasped hands all the way to the back of your neck.

Repetitions: 1

Underarm Stretch

The purpose of this exercise is to stretch your underarm and the muscles in the back of your affected arm. As with the clasp-lift stretch, the underarm stretch should be done only after your drains are out or (if you have no drains) after the second week.

Position: Stand facing a wall.

Motion: Lift your affected arm as far as possible and lay your palm flat against the wall. Lean forward until you feel a stretch in your underarm area. Hold that position for 15 seconds. Return to an upright position and lower your arm. Do this stretch only once daily. Over time, you'll note improvement in your ability to stretch, and you can stand farther from the wall to start.

Repetitions: 1

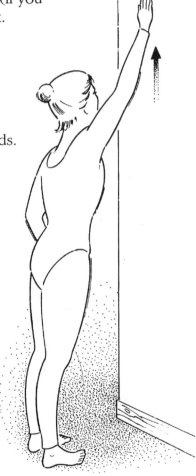

Upper Torso Stretches

Corner Stretches

To help stretch your chest muscles, you'll want to do corner stretches daily, beginning with the third week. This exercise should never be done when drains are in place.

Position: Stand facing the corner of the room.

Motion: With bent elbows, place the palms of your hands against each side of the corner, so your forearms touch the walls and your elbows are at shoulder level.

Slowly lean forward, moving your chest toward the corner. Keep your elbows at shoulder level and your forearms flat against the wall as you lean in. You will feel the stretch across your chest. Hold this position for 15 seconds. Do this stretch only once daily.

Repetitions: 1

Weightlifting Exercises

Beginning in the third week and continuing throughout your recovery, some gentle weightlifting exercises will help build your arm muscles, keep them strong, and reduce your risk for *lymphedema*, a potentially chronic swelling caused by a collection of excess lymph fluid.

When all drains are removed, and you have started stretching on a daily basis, you should be ready to begin the slightly more strenuous weightlifting exercises, listed in the pages ahead. To do them, you will need small weights, ranging in size from one pound to five pounds. You may purchase them in any fitness or sports store.

Alternatively (if you don't want to buy weights), you can start out using some one-pound canned goods. Later, as you build up to higher weights, partially-filled, plastic water jugs can be substituted for weights.

Weightlifting exercises take about ten minutes to do and should be repeated every other day. You can combine or alternate them with stretching exercises. To avoid injury or over-straining when exercising with weights, be sure to follow these guidelines:

- Use weights weighing five pounds or less. If you have previously used heavier weights and think you may be able to resume your previous routine, ask your hospital physical therapist for instruction.
- Perform these exercises only once a day, and never do them two days in a row. You'll be putting your muscles under some stress, and they need time to repair themselves.
- Stand erect in front of a mirror to check your form.

- Breathe correctly. Exhale with the effort, when you are lifting the weight. Inhale when you lower the weight and relax the muscle.

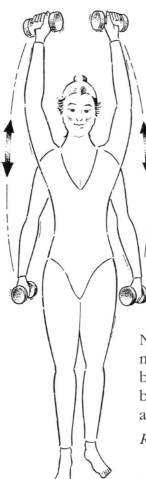

Shoulder Flexion

This weight-lifting exercise works the deltoid muscle, which covers the upper part of your shoulder. This is the muscle flexed when you lift your arm overhead.

Position: Stand with your arms by your sides, holding weights comfortably in your hands. Your hands should be in a natural position, with the weights parallel to the floor.

Motion: Raise both arms evenly in front of your body, until both hands are directly overhead. As you perform this motion, keep your arms straight, and exhale.

Now lower your arms, reversing the same motion. Keep your arms straight as you bring them down directly in front of your body. Inhale as you slowly lower both arms.

Repetitions: 10

Biceps Curl

The biceps are upper-arm muscles that help you lift your lower arm and hand. The biceps curl will help to return normal strength to that muscle.

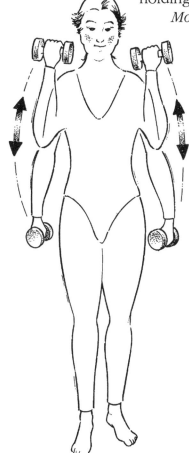

Position: Stand with your arms by your sides, holding a weight in each hand.

Motion: Bend your arms and lift them, bringing your hands (with the weights) as close to your shoulders as possible. Exhale as you perform this motion. Slowly return your hands and arms to the starting position. Inhale.

Repetitions: 10

Arm Extension

This exercise strengthens the triceps muscle, which is under your upper arm, directly opposite the biceps. It's the muscle that helps you straighten the arm.

Position: Lie on your back on a mat or carpet, with your arms by your sides. Begin with a weight in your affected hand. Lift your lower arm from the floor by bending your elbow and raising the weight until your lower arm is perpendicular to the floor. Hold the upper part of your weight-bearing arm with your opposite hand to steady your arm during the entire exercise.

Motion: Lift your whole arm from the floor, keeping the elbow bent, bringing the weight toward your shoulder until your elbow points toward the ceiling. Slowly straighten the arm until it is fully extended and your hand points toward the ceiling. Hold it for a few seconds. Exhale as you perform this motion. Slowly bring the weight toward your shoulder until your elbow points towards the ceiling. Inhale as you do so.

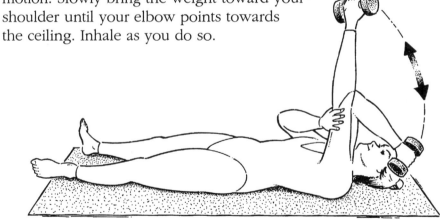

Repetitions: 10 on each side

Include a Daily Walking Program

In addition to stretching and lifting light weights, walking every day will not only give you more energy, it also will help your emotional and physical recovery. In fact, research has shown that a daily walk increases energy levels and helps elevate one's mood. It's often recommended as a treatment for mild to moderate depression.

The goal is a daily thirty-minute walk, but you don't have to walk the full thirty minutes your first day out. You might want to start with one or two five-minute walks every day, then gradually lengthen your walking time. If it's impractical to spend half an hour walking, try for three ten-minute walks daily. As you increase the duration of your walks, increase the pace as well.

The most beneficial kind of walking is continuous. Stop-and-go activities—such as running errands, housework, even gardening—are likely to make you more tired, while continuous walking actually makes you feel more energetic.

Resuming Your Normal Activities

In six weeks your chest muscle will have healed completely. With daily stretching and strength training three times a week, you should regain your full arm mobility and strength. Normally, that's when you can

---

Benefits of a Daily Walk

- Improves energy
- Helps mental functioning
- Improves bone density, reducing the risk of osteoporosis
- Exercises your heart and lungs, reducing your risk of heart disease
- Improves your mood
- Reduces stress
- Helps you sleep better at night
- Reduces the number and intensity of hot flashes and night sweats
- Regularizes bowel movements
- Helps with weight loss
- Reduces the risk of lymphedema
- Enhances your immune system

resume sports that you enjoyed before surgery, such as golf, tennis, swimming, or running. Of course, your surgeon needs to give you the okay before you resume aerobic exercise or return to a customary workout routine.

If you start chemotherapy—which usually begins three to four weeks after surgery—you'll probably experience the common, temporary side effect of fatigue. So you may find that you don't have the stamina for strenuous exercise. Check with your doctors and nurses about continuing your exercise program.

3

Nutrition: A Guide to Healthful Eating

Good nutrition is essential for good health. It is especially important to eat health-promoting foods when your body is recovering from surgery or treatment for cancer. A nutrient-rich diet helps you maintain your strength and prevents body tissue from breaking down. It also helps rebuild tissues that may be harmed during chemotherapy or radiation treatments.

In addition to helping you recover from surgery, good nutrition *may* also help combat cancer. Right now, there is not enough scientific evidence to prove that specific foods cause cancer or that others prevent it, but comprehensive studies by major health organizations have published nutritional guidelines, which if followed, may lower one's risk of cancer.

An "Anti-Cancer" Diet

Nutritional guidelines from both the American Institute for Cancer Research and the American Cancer Society suggest that a cancer-fighting food plan should include a variety of plant-based foods—at least five servings of fruits and vegetables daily, along with beans, nuts, seeds, and whole grains. Red meats, if eaten at all, should be limited to less than three ounces daily. Fish and skinless poultry are recommended in place of red meat.

Why a diet rich in plant-based foods? These foods contain compounds called *phytonutrients* (plant nutrients) that seem to boost the body's natural defenses against *carcinogens*—that is, cancer-causing substances. In populations where people depend on plant-based diets, their intake of phytonutrients seems to combat carcinogens and help protect body cells from damage. Thus, cancer risk is reduced.

There are many ways you can increase the proportion of phytonutrients in your diet without making radical lifestyle changes. You don't need to go out of your way to do so. In fact, your best resource is no farther away than your nearest supermarket. There is, however, one particular food that is generally under-utilized in the American diet, and it seems to provide special benefits as a cancer fighter.

That food is soy.

The Japanese Diet—A Special Case

For some time, medical researchers have been intrigued by studies showing that Japanese women, whose diets are high in soy, have a significantly lower risk of getting breast cancer than American women. Natural products made from soybeans include such foods as soymilk, tofu, tempeh, edamame (whole green soybean), and soy nut (baked soybean), all of which are prominent in the traditional Japanese diet. The incidence of breast cancer among Japanese women is 5 per 100,000. America's rate, by contrast, is 22.4 per 100,000. A Japanese woman has about one-fourth the risk of getting breast cancer as an American woman.

It is important to keep in mind that the "traditional" Japanese diet also includes many other plant-based foods—among them, seaweed and Shiitake mushrooms (which most Americans don't eat). Their diet also includes a high proportion of fish, while Americans tend to eat more meat. Japanese women have low consumption of alcohol, and they ingest almost no processed foods and *hydrogenated oils*, those used in such foods as commercially baked goods. But even when these differences are taken into account, researchers think it's likely that soybeans have a special component that helps reduce breast cancer risk.

Recommended Sources of Carbohydrates

Current nutritional guidelines suggest that most Americans should be getting more vegetables, fruits, and whole grains in their diets. All these foods contain "complex carbohydrates." When you eat them, you unlock rich sources of vitamins and minerals that help protect your body cells and improve the way your organs function.

Unprocessed fruits, vegetables, grains, and beans offer other benefits. These foods are high in fiber. Studies have shown that groups of people on high-fiber diets tend to have a lower incidence of colon cancer, heart disease, and other health problems than people who live on low-fiber diets.

Cruciferous Vegetables

Studies have consistently found that people who eat cruciferous vegetables—members of the "cabbage family"—have a lower risk of cancer, particularly breast cancer. The compound in

Cruciferous Vegetables
with Indole-3 Carbinol

- Bok choy
- Broccoli
- Brussels Sprouts
- Cabbage
- Radish
- Kale
- Mustard seed
- Rutabaga
- Turnip
- Watercress

these vegetables that seems to be the chief cancer fighter is indole-3 carbinol.

Indole-3 carbinol and other compounds stimulate detoxification in the body—that is, they remove and/or deactivate harmful substances from the body that can cause cell damage. Numerous animal and cell culture studies show that indole-3 is a potent antagonist of breast cancer cells.

Carbohydrate Sources to Avoid

When you eat simple carbohydrates such as—white bread, pasta, white rice, packaged cereals, rice cakes, crackers, cookies, and cakes—you're missing the benefits you get from nutrient-rich foods. Packaged and processed foods contribute little to your health, and many are harmful to the extent that they cause weight gain and blood sugar problems.

How so? Once digested, these foods become sugar in the body and stimulate the production of insulin. In turn, the body converts the sugar into fat and stores it, which adds to your supply of body fat. Our fat makes and stores estrogen, and studies show that being overweight increases the risk of recurrence if your cancer is estrogen positive. In addition, we do know that obesity increases our risks for a variety of many other diseases, particularly heart disease and adult onset (type-2) diabetes.

So it's important to think about the carbohydrates you choose. When you have an apple for a snack instead of crackers or cookies, for instance, you're giving your body the nutrient-rich reward of complex carbohydrates rather than "empty" calories that raise your blood-sugar levels and contribute to weight gain.

Recommended Sources of Protein

Protein is essential to repair tissue damage from surgery, chemotherapy, and radiation therapy, and it should be part of your diet every day. Protein can be found in both plant and animal food sources. Although many people think of red meat as a prime source of protein, there are other, more healthful sources as well. Beans, fish, nuts, and non-fat dairy products are among the other good sources.

Many studies have shown that vegetarians have a lower rate of all kinds of cancers and most diseases (heart disease, diabetes, osteoporosis) compared to people who eat a lot of red meat and poultry. Soybeans, black beans, garbanzo beans, red beans, and kidney beans are sources of plant protein.

> **Fish High in Omega-3 Fats**
> - Mackerel, Atlantic
> - Trout, lake
> - Herring, Atlantic
> - Tuna, Albacore
> - Salmon, Atlantic

In addition to being good sources of protein, beans have a number of other benefits. They are high in fiber and contain no saturated fat (so they do not increase your risk of heart disease). Plus, they are inexpensive and easy to prepare.

Protein from Fish

In countries where people eat a lot of deep-water and cold-water fish, the populations usually have a decreased incidence of both cancer and heart disease. Fish is an excellent source of protein. It also has a kind of fat called omega-3 that seems to help as a cancer-fighting agent.

35

Fish has another benefit. It is also rich in vitamin D, a nutrient that researchers have found helps ward off breast cancer in post-menopausal women. If you enjoy eating fish, two or three servings per week is recommended.

Protein from Dairy Products

Milk, cheese, yogurt, and many other dairy products are good sources of protein, but these foods are usually high in saturated fat. However, you can take advantage of the availability of nonfat and low-fat dairy products found on most supermarket shelves. By choosing skim milk over whole milk, for instance, you get the same amount of protein without any fat content. You can also find nonfat or low-fat cheeses and yogurts that have good protein content, with very little or no saturated fat which contributes to weight gain, diabetes, and heart disease.

Meats in Moderation

Most of us find that meats such as steak, hamburger, and chicken are hard to give up. The solution is to cut back on portion size. For a nutritional balance and plenty of protein, all you need are three ounces (after cooking) of red meat or poultry once a day. That serving is just about the size of a deck of cards. If you're accustomed to more than that, the reduced portion may look small. But if you load up the rest of your plate with the recommended servings of plant foods, you'll be getting a filling and tasty meal that's much more healthful.

A Warning about Grilled Meat

Grilled meats including poultry and fish, may be particularly harmful to health. Studies show that if you barbecue, broil, or pan-fry meat at high heat, the cooking process introduces a substance called *heterocyclic amines*. These substances are thought to contribute to cancer development. In animal studies, scientists have learned that heterocyclic amines damage the genetic material inside cells and induce tumors.

Meats that are boiled, stewed, or poached have fewer harmful substances, particularly if the meat is cooked rare to medium. If you definitely like grilling and you want to reduce the presence of the carcinogenic substances, you can microwave meat or poultry for two to five minutes before putting it on the grill. That releases juices that contain precursors of heterocyclic amines. (Be sure to discard the juice.) Or you can marinate the meat before grilling in a marinade that has lots of lemon or lime juice. The marinade reduces the presence of carcinogens.

Recommended Sources of Fat

Fat is often misunderstood. For years, doctors and nutritionists advocated low-fat diets to help us lose weight and improve our blood cholesterol levels. This point is well taken since most of us consume too much fat. However, we all need *some* fat as part of good nutrition. We can't live without it. Among other things, fats keep our cell membranes fluid and flexible. They promote growth of cells, blood vessels, and nerves, and they keep skin and other tissues lubricated.

However, not all fats are alike. There are several types of fats, some good for us, others bad for us. The good fats are *unsaturated fats*, and there are two categories of these:

- **Polyunsaturated fats**: found in fish and plant sources such as vegetable oils, nuts and seeds.
- **Monounsaturated fats**: found in oils such as canola, and olive.

Particularly desirable polyunsaturated fats are those found in the cold-water fish like tuna and salmon—that is, omega-3 fats, an essential fatty acid. Studies have shown that the omega-3s improve the ratio of the so-called "good cholesterol" (HDL) to "bad cholesterol" (LDL), so they benefit arterial health.

Although cold-water fish are a prime source of omega-3 fats, there are others as well. Other good plant sources include flaxseed, soybeans, walnuts, oat germ, raw spinach, wheat germ, and raw broccoli.

Fats to Avoid

In the last thirty years consumers have increased their consumption of man-made fats. The increased consumption of bad fats has, no doubt, contributed to the incidence of heart disease. And, some research suggests that too much fat in the diet may contribute to the development of cancer. The types of "bad fats" include:

> **Saturated fats**: mainly found in animal fats, whole-milk products, and some plant foods, including coconut and coconut oil, palm oil, and palm kernel oil.

> **Trans fats**: this fat, which acts like a saturated fat, is produced by heating vegetable oil to a solid state to extend the shelf life of food products. This process is known as hydrogenation. The more solid the fat, the more *trans fats*. These *hydrogenated fats* are found in commercially prepared baked goods, margarine, snack foods, and processed foods. Commercially fried foods, such as French fries, are high in trans fats.

Another fat, omega-6 fats, are those that come from such foods as vegetable oils and the meat of grain fed animals. Too much of these fats can lead to increased blood clotting and constricting of blood vessels, leading to increased risk of heart disease and stroke and possibly cancer. Although no absolute link between omega-6 fats and breast cancer has been proved, some research shows that women with breast cancer have a higher consumption of "bad fats." The western diet contains up to twenty times as much omega-6 as omega-3 fats or a 20:0 ratio. The ratio should be closer to 4:1. The American Institute for Cancer Research recommends cutting back on consumption of omega-6 fats. In short, women interested in breast cancer prevention would want to reduce consumption of harmful fats found in vegetable oils, margarines, and fried or packaged fast foods. Read labels before you buy packaged foods. Avoid products that contain "hydrogenated" or "partially hydrogenated" oils. Many "diet" foods or processed foods are loaded with these kinds of harmful fats.

Oils with Omega-6 Fats
• Corn oil
• Safflower oil
• Sunflower oil
• Peanut oil
• Cottonseed oil
• Grapeseed oil
• Sesame oil

Recommended Beverages

Good hydration is an essential to every cell in your body. It's especially important to drink a lot of water when you are undergoing chemotherapy or radiation therapy. When you drink plenty of liquids, you help flush waste and toxins from your body.

Try to drink eight to ten eight-ounce glasses of hydrating liquids a day. In addition to water, other recommended liquids include diluted fruit juice, herbal tea, soy milk, and non-caffeinated sodas. Fruits, particularly watermelon, are hydrating, too.

Beverages to Avoid

Surprisingly enough, there are some beverages that actually contribute to *dehydration* rather than helping to restore fluids to your system. Drinks that contain caffeine or alcohol are diuretics. They stimulate removal of water from the body. And when you lose fluids, your body is depleted of crucial nutrients, including water-soluble vitamins (such as vitamin C) and minerals (such as calcium). As a rule of thumb, you need to drink at least two glasses of water to compensate for every cup of coffee or glass of wine you drink. If you have two cups of coffee in the morning, for instance, you should try to drink four glasses of water, too.

There's an easy way to tell if you are getting dehydrated. Look at your urine. If it's dark yellow, you probably need to get more water and other liquids in your diet. Also, poor hydration contributes to fatigue. So if you often feel tired, that may be another indication that you're not getting enough hydrating liquids during the day.

What about Alcohol?

A number of studies suggest that people who consume one glass of alcohol a day have an increased risk of breast cancer. On the other hand, wine (especially red wine) contains an ingredient called *resveratrol*, which is considered an anti-cancer agent.

If you enjoy drinking a glass of wine with your family or friends, do so in moderation. For women, the recommendation is less than one serving of an alcoholic drink per day. A serving is defined as 5 ounces of wine, 12 ounces of regular beer, or 1.5 ounces of 80-proof distilled spirits.

As for resveratrol, there are some ways to get this cancer-fighting ingredient without drinking red wine. It is also found in red grapes and in grape juice. In fact, red wine might not be the best source of this ingredient. Once the wine bottle is opened, resveratrol evaporates within twenty-four hours.

4

Coping Emotionally

In the Chinese language, the character representing the word "crisis" is a combination of two symbols, one for danger and the other for opportunity. Many breast cancer patients would say this symbol is a fitting description of a serious illness—they are frightened, but are also given the opportunity to evaluate what is really important in life. In fact, many women describe breast cancer as both the worst thing and the best thing that has ever happened to them.

For someone who has just received a cancer diagnosis, it may be impossible to imagine that this could possibly be the "best" of anything. You are immediately confronted with emotional and physical challenges that may be greater than anything you've dealt with before. How could there possibly be anything positive in this experience? But women often find they have many positive experiences during the healing—physically and emotionally—that follows a mastectomy.

Getting in Touch with Self

As we slow down and focus on our lives, we can explore our own needs and desires, and connect more with others for emotional and practical support. This gives us an opportunity to deepen relationships with others while developing a better understanding of ourselves. We can create more intimate and satisfying relationships. And, often, we have a chance to deepen our spirituality. A feeling of connection with a higher power, or a sense of connection with the universe, may be awakened. In times like these we learn that the human spirit has amazing strength, resilience, and capacity to overcome suffering.

As you travel the path of recovery from cancer, you'll experience strong and contradictory emotions. You may feel hopeful one moment and scared the next. You may have some days when you feel completely calm and composed, followed by others when you're angry—at yourself, at God, at your doctors, and even at those you love.

Each woman has her own way of coping with a difficult situation. Some have easy access to their feelings and readily express themselves. Others are more reserved and private. Some women throw themselves into the cancer experience, want to know everything, and frequently talk about it. Others avoid the subject and seek distractions.

There is no right or wrong way to cope. Your emotional recovery lies in your ability to make your own needs and feelings your top priority. And, there are a number of steps you can take to enhance your recovery process.

Relationships with Your Doctors

When you were first diagnosed with cancer, you may have felt like you had lost control of your body and your life. Many women find that by having a good relationship with doctors, they feel more in control and also more committed to treatment.

If you don't have an open relationship with your doctors, you can still develop one. It's never too late to start expressing your concerns or asking questions. You may feel reluctant to ask questions. But if you can overcome that reluctance and gather as much information as possible about what lies ahead, you'll reduce your anxiety.

As you continue to see your surgeon or other doctors during the course of treatment, write down your questions and concerns as you think of them. Take the list with you when you visit doctors, therapists, or other health care professionals. Remember, there is no such thing as a "silly" or "dumb" question.

Do you find it difficult to remember what was said in discussions with your doctors? You can take notes, of course, but your mind may wander as you try to deal with the implications of what you're hearing. Why not ask your partner, a family member, or a friend to go along to your next visit? Afterward, the two of you can review what was said and make sure your questions were answered.

Make a List of Priorities

With surgery behind you, what do you need now and in the days ahead? Take time to decide what is really important right now. Make a list of the activities and responsibilities you can handle. Make another list of those that are physically and emotionally draining. How many obligations can you cancel? Which items can other people take care of? Jot down the names of friends, family members, or co-workers who can help you.

Every day, you need to do at least one activity that makes you feel good and that gives you pleasure. What brings you joy? Think of the simple and attainable pleasures that are within reach—walking in the park, sitting on your porch watching a sunset or the night sky, scratching your dog behind the ears or playing with your cat, listening to favorite music, or relaxing in a warm bath. Each day, take some time to enjoy the activities that are most comforting and make you feel happy to be alive.

Asking for Support

Many women are used to putting other people's needs—those of children, partner, family, friends and co-workers—ahead of their own. If that describes you, then you'll probably find it difficult to ask others for help. Yet it's important to learn to ask, even if you feel awkward or guilty at first. To take care of yourself, you have to reach out to other people who can provide support.

Often, loved ones, even partners, would like to help but are not sure what to say or do. Keep in mind that they, too, may be frightened and worried. They need your help in letting them know *how* they can help.

It's okay to tell them what you need. For example, sometimes all you need is for someone who cares about you to *just be there*—to sit with you, to listen, to let you cry.

Or maybe you need to be touched. Having your hand held, or hugging somebody, can be very healing. The direct approach is the best. It's fine to say, "Would you hold my hand?" Or "I need a hug!" Right away, the other person will stop wondering what to do next or how to help.

At other times, you'll need to be cheered up or distracted. You can invite others to share a meal, a cup of tea, or a laugh. A friend or family member can accompany you on a nature walk, go with you to service, sit with you in a concert, or pray with you.

With a simple, direct invitation, let the other person know that you'd like companionship.

Spouses, family members, and friends can also provide practical assistance to help you conserve your energy. Some people feel more comfortable showing their support by "doing" rather than talking or listening. Ask them to help you with meals. Ask them to run errands, to care for your children, to drive you to appointments.

Be as specific as possible. If someone has offered to make a meal, for instance, let them know about your or your family's favorite foods, and express your appreciation for the offer. If others offer to help take care of the children, suggest some activities that the kids enjoy.

Protect Yourself by Setting Boundaries

Not everyone is able to give you the support and the understanding you need in the way you need it. Some of your co-workers, friends, and even family, no matter how well-meaning, might say things that make you feel worse rather than better.

When others offer advice you don't feel you need, you may need to protect yourself by setting boundaries. You might politely say, "Thank you for your interest, but I'd rather not discuss this right now." Or, "I know that you are trying to be helpful and I so appreciate that, but I would prefer to get my information and treatment recommendations from my doctors." This approach will not only spare their feelings, but more importantly, spare *you* needless stress and heartache.

Though family and friends want frequent updates, how can you keep everyone advised of your progress all the time? You may start to feel overwhelmed with constant telephone calls from loved ones asking how the treatments are going and how you're feeling. There are a number of ways to handle the updates, depending on your preference. Do you like to tell as many people as possible, or would you rather be more private about your health and your feelings? The following approaches can help conserve your physical and emotional energy:

- Ask one, designated person whom you trust to keep others informed.
- Use a telephone answering machine to screen your calls. When you don't have the desire or the energy to return calls, record a message that says, "Thanks for calling. I am a little tired, so I'll probably not get back to you right away. But I would love to hear your message. Please keep it under three minutes."
- E-mails, particularly group e-mails, can be an efficient and great way to keep in touch with family and friends. If you don't enjoy e-mailing, a family member or a friend can take care of this for you.

When People Pull Away

Sometimes, a close friend or relative pulls away and becomes cold and distant. In extreme cases, the person may literally disappear from your life with no clear explanation. This often comes as a shock. Such an absence may be very painful to you.

Trying to understand *why* people do this can be exhausting and frustrating. But it's important to remember that these people are not rejecting you personally. For whatever reason, they have personal issues that have very little to do with you. Perhaps their own fears of cancer, or other fears about personal health, create feelings they can't tolerate in themselves.

If this happens, surround yourself with those who can be truly supportive. You can decide some other time whether you want to "leave the door open" for the return of someone who has not been supportive. But right now, you need people who are dependable.

Talking to Your Children

You may be tempted to protect your children, and maybe yourself, by not telling them about having had a mastectomy. But children can sense when something is wrong, even when they're very young. It's better to be honest with them. Tell them the truth, simply and in a manner and language appropriate to their age level.

How do you know what is age appropriate and what they need to know? You'll find out by encouraging questions from them. When they ask, give them the information they ask for, but don't offer more until they ask again. Often, children absorb stressful information in stages. After they have time to internalize the information you've given them, they will ask more questions when they are ready.

Typically when children are feeling scared and stressed, they regress, acting more like children—more "babyish," less responsible. They worry that something will happen to you and that you will go away. It will help them if they can maintain their normal routines and activities as much as possible. This helps children feel secure in the knowledge that everything is okay.

Talking to Your Mate

A diagnosis of cancer can indeed strengthen the love in a relationship. Studies consistently show that the experience of going through cancer together strengthens good marriages and relationships. The process of healing brings more intimacy to a relationship and can bring couples closer together. On the other hand, if you are in an emotionally-strained relationship, it may not be able to withstand the emotional test. Your own anger, or your partner's, may surface in unanticipated ways. In a deeply troubled marriage or an abusive relationship, cancer can be a catalyst for change, liberating you and your children to create a healthier and safer life.

Hopefully, your relationship is already a strong one and your mate is at your side to support you through your recovery. Even then, communication is important. Your needs will have changed, and your mate may not always be readily aware of what they are. Again, it's important to ask for what you need.

It's important, too, to realize what and how your mate is able to give. For example, a mate who is the "silent type," probably won't become a talker after your cancer diagnosis. Someone, who is not handy with homemaking tasks, may not be able to take over the cooking and the house cleaning. All the same, your partner can learn new ways to help you, if you express what you need to feel safe and protected. You, in turn, can accept your partner's help graciously and without criticism. Although your partner may not load the dishwasher or do the laundry just the way you like it done, your appreciation for what is offered will likely encourage further participation.

One way to ask for support is by asking your partner to accompany you when you visit your doctors. Doctors' visits are an opportunity for your partner to get questions answered as well.

If you have children, encourage your partner to spend extra time with them. This not only strengthens the relationship between your mate and the children, it also makes the children feel more secure. Their outings give you a chance for time alone, if you need it.

If you feel you're having trouble communicating with your partner, or need help coping with the changes in your life and relationship, talk to your partner about seeing a marriage counselor. Often, just a few sessions can get you both on the right path of love and support.

Physical and Sexual Intimacy

Women consistently express an awareness that femininity, womanhood, and sexuality are much more than having breasts. But even so, a woman who has gone through a mastectomy may feel insecure about her new body.

In the beginning, you may not feel the need or be ready for sexual intimacy, but you probably find comfort in being touched and hugged. It's very important to let your partner know that you need that kind of warm, physical contact. Sometimes even without noticing it, couples drift apart physically.

If you notice that you and your partner have less physical contact than you used to, make an effort to start touching again. Holding hands, asking for or giving a hug, stroking an arm or back is a powerful intimate exchange for both you and your partner.

Sometimes a neck or back massage is very comforting. The intimate experience can bring pleasure to both of you. Don't hesitate to ask for a massage. To make the experience more comfortable, you can either lie on your unaffected side or sit up. Your partner can enhance the massage by using lotion or oil. It doesn't have to be an energetic massage. Just a gentle back-rub or neck-rub can be soothing—and the touching will bring you closer emotionally as well.

Resuming Sexual Relations

If you and your partner had a rich sexual life before your surgery, try to resume it again as soon as possible. Making love is life affirming. It gives you pleasure, and brings you closer together.

You may find that both you and your partner have less interest in sex than you did before your mastectomy. This is quite common. The stress of diagnosis, surgery, and possible treatment, along with the many strong emotions you're probably feeling, may reduce sexual desire.

If so, it's important to talk about those feelings. If you don't discuss those feelings there is the potential for misunderstanding and hurt feelings. But, as with all other aspects of your emotional recovery, it's important for you to be honest with yourself about your needs, concerns, and fears. Talk with your partner about them. It may help if you can start these conversations.

Physical Comfort and Sexual Intimacy

Sometimes, partners assume that you shouldn't have sex for some time after surgery. The fear that lovemaking will hurt you may make your partner hesitant. Women often misinterpret this as rejection. You can prevent this potential misunderstanding by talking frankly. Reassure your partner that lovemaking won't harm your incision and that it isn't bad for your health. Your partner can reassure you that you are still loved and desired.

Whenever you and your partner feel ready to have sexual relations, here are some suggestions:

- Wear something that makes you feel comfortable and desirable.
- Encourage your partner to look at your incision or your reconstructed breast and also to touch it. This helps both of you get comfortable with the new you. Let your partner know how it feels when your incision and chest are touched. Those areas may be tender, numb, or particularly sensitive to touch, and your partner needs to be aware of that. Some women don't enjoy having the area over the incision caressed; others do. It's important to let your partner know what feels good and what doesn't.
- Remember, there is no right or wrong position for having sex. Whatever position is comfortable for you is "right."
- Protect your incision or reconstructed breast if you need to do so to relax. Try lying on your back with your unaffected arm crossed protectively over the incision or reconstructed breast and your hand resting on your affected shoulder. Alternatively, you can place a small pillow under your arm, or over your chest or tummy for protection. If you feel safer this way, it will be easier to enjoy sex.
- To make intercourse more comfortable, you can select from a number of good, non-prescription products that provide vaginal lubrication. Tamoxifen or chemotherapy can cause vaginal dryness, which makes intercourse uncomfortable.

Single Women and Sexual Intimacy

If you are a single woman without a partner, you may have some special concerns about emotional and physical intimacy. You may worry about dating and starting a new romantic relationship. You may also have concerns about when and how to tell a new friend or potential lover that you have had breast surgery.

Most single women find it can be helpful to talk to *other* single women who have had breast cancer. A breast cancer support group is a good place to find out how they've coped. Ask your hospital social worker, doctors, nurses—and look in the Resource section of this book—for groups that can put you in touch with other single women who have had a mastectomy.

Overcoming Depression

It is perfectly normal to feel sad and to cry. You'll probably feel better after a good cry. However, if you feel sad all the time, you may be suffering from clinical depression.

Clinical depression is a label for a range of symptoms that are quite common, particularly among people who have experienced serious illness. An estimated twenty-three percent of breast cancer patients suffer from clinical depression after surgery. Receiving proper treatment—often with a combination of counseling and medications—can help you feel much better.

There are compelling reasons to treat clinical depression. Left untreated, it can interfere with physical and emotional recovery. But how do you know the difference between sadness and depression?

If you are feeling several of the following symptoms for more than two weeks, you may have clinical depression. Ask yourself: "Does this describe the way I've been feeling recently?"

- Constant and excessive feelings of worthlessness, hopelessness, guilt, shame and/or fear
- Disinterest in food, or excessive eating
- Inability to sleep, or sleeping too much
- Constant jitters or nervousness
- Not feeling pleasure; losing interest in things that used to interest you
- A loss of libido (losing interest in sex)
- Suicidal thoughts

If it seems as if you're having a lot of these symptoms, start by seeing a mental health professional who can do an evaluation and recommend treatment. In addition to individual counseling with a therapist (usually a psychiatrist, psychologist, or clinical social worker), your treatment might include a combination of the following:

- Exercise
- Stress reduction techniques
- Spiritual counseling
- A support group
- Medications

Should You Take Antidepressants?

Being depressed changes your brain chemistry, and sometimes the best thing you can do is to take medication. Studies have shown that only two percent of cancer patients who suffer from depression receive medication. Probably many more could be helped. Talking with a psychiatrist, a doctor that specializes in mental health and medications can help you.

Many women who resist taking antidepressants seem to believe that the medication will make them feel happy all the time. That leads to the fear that the medication will have a dulling effect and they won't be able to deal with sad and painful feelings. This concern is unwarranted. Antidepressants don't make you feel instantly happy, buoyant, or elated. Rather, they diminish your depression, so that you actually are better able to deal with your feelings. None of them create the feelings of euphoria that people get from recreational drugs.

How Antidepressants Work

Since depression is associated with a chemical imbalance in the brain, antidepressants come to the rescue by fine-tuning brain chemistry. The "messengers" that carry signals from one brain cell to another are called *neurotransmitters*. When neurotransmitters are out of balance, there's a risk of depression.

Commonly prescribed antidepressants include:
- Paxil (Paroxetine)
- Prozac (Fluoxetine)
- Zoloft (Sertraline)
- Celexa (Citalopram)
- Effexor (Venlafaxine)
- Serzone (Nefazadone)
- Remeron (Mirtazapine)
- Wellbutrin (Bupropion)

Antidepressants, some more than others, have possible side effects. These include headache, anxiety, flushing, difficulty falling asleep, feeling "jittery," problems with sexual functioning, loss of appetite, upset stomach, dizziness, and tremors. If you have problems with these or any other medication, let your psychiatrist know. The side effects often diminish as you continue taking them. Your doctor might recommend switching to another medication that won't affect you the same way.

Keep in mind that it may take two to four weeks before antidepressants deliver their full therapeutic benefits.

Join a Support Group

After cancer surgery, you may feel different, isolated, and alone. A support group offers understanding, strength, and companionship. Surprisingly enough, you'll find humor, too—moments of belly-splitting laughter. It's such a relief to discover that you are not alone.

When you hear other women expressing feelings similar to yours, you realize that those feelings are normal and part of the healing process. In a support group, you have a safe place to express feelings that you can't or won't share with family or friends. Whether you have family or not, your breast cancer support group becomes a "family" of special friends.

Before attending a meeting, call the facilitator. By getting to know one person before you go, you'll feel more comfortable when you first attend. If you're not sure whether you really want to join a particular group, be sure to attend at least two meetings before you decide. Each support group has its own personality, uniquely defined by the women who participate and by the facilitator, and it takes a while to decide whether the group you visit will be a good fit. If, after a couple of meetings, you decide the group doesn't feel right, don't be discouraged. Just try another one. It's worth it. Many women say that finding a comfortable support group, and staying with it, has been vital in their emotional recovery.

Another alternative is to get in touch with another woman who has had a mastectomy. While her experience will not be exactly the same as yours, there is much you can share in one-to-one conversations.

Seek Spiritual Support

Spirituality and prayer can be a great source of comfort, strength, and healing. But for some women, a diagnosis of cancer marks the beginning of a spiritual crisis. Even if you have a strong spiritual life, you may begin to question everything you believe in. Feelings of betrayal are common. You may wonder, "Why is God punishing me?" For someone who has held to a strong faith all her life, spiritual alienation can be hard to bear.

If you have previously found comfort in spirituality, you may be ashamed about your doubts. There is no reason to hide these feelings. They are common. But don't give up on trying to find spiritual guidance. A spiritual counselor will understand your distress and, even if you feel shaken in your faith, might help you regain your spiritual balance.

Some women find their spirituality is reawakened. They may start to rethink their values, examining what is really important in life. They may rekindle relationships and develop greater intimacy. They may be inspired by acts of kindness and love.

If you are experiencing a spiritual awakening, take this opportunity to deepen it. Seek spiritual counseling, practice yoga, join a congregation, join a choir, or engage in regular prayer or meditation.

At the End of Treatment

After your surgery and any subsequent treatments, you may actually feel more fragile. It's reassuring to realize that your body is healing, but your emotions may still be raw. When you finish treatment, it's particularly important to ask for and receive emotional support.

During treatment, you are focusing on making decisions and recovering physically. You also felt protected because you were being seen frequently by your doctors. And, frankly, during treatment, most people are very sympathetic. They are compassionate when they see that you are in pain or have less energy. But once treatment is over and you start looking and acting like your old self, your loved ones may assume that everything is just as it was before. They may become less supportive and even impatient, expecting you to "get on with your life." But, once you have been diagnosed with breast cancer, *you* know your life will never be the same.

Hopefully, the experience of breast cancer will remind you to live each day to the fullest. And each day, it may be helpful to remind yourself that you are not alone. More than two million women in the United States are living with breast cancer. These women have found, in themselves and through others, the strength and resources to recover and heal. You are part of this community of survivors.

5

Breast Forms and Undergarments

If you chose not to have breast reconstruction, you may have given some thought to breast forms. Most women are very pleased with them. They find the forms restore their shape and reassures them that they look natural in their clothes.

You may wear a light-weight temporary breast form right after your surgery; however, you'll need to ask your surgeon when you can start wearing a permanent form, also known as a *prosthesis*. Usually, you need to wait six to eight weeks after your surgery, allowing time for the swelling to resolve.

It is important that your permanent breast form be the appropriate size. It is equally important that your bra fits correctly. You may be able to use your current bra, but many women have never worn the correct bra size. Why? Because they were never professionally fitted for one. Now, the correct fit is important for both your comfort and health.

Temporary Breast Forms

Temporary forms should be made of a soft, lightweight material. You can choose from various kinds of temporary forms in a post-mastectomy boutique or a medical supply store. Or you can make your own form by using a foam rubber or a cloth-covered shoulder pad.

Some special camisoles come with temporary breast forms. Or you can simply use a safety pin to attach a temporary form to your own camisole, undershirt, or slip. As soon as it's comfortable to wear a bra, you can pin the breast form into your bra cup. If the shoulder pad rides up in your bra, sew drapery weights into your breast form to keep your bra in place.

Another option, once you begin wearing a bra, is to place lamb's wool in your bra cup. The lamb's wool is especially nice because it is soft, absorbent, and comfortable. Lamb's wool can be purchased at your pharmacy.

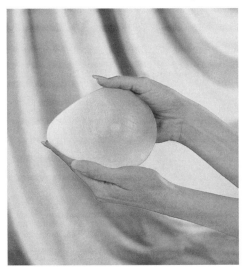

Permanent breast forms are made with silicone gel. Photo courtesy of Amoena.

Permanent Breast Forms

A permanent breast form is made of durable silicone gel with a polyurethane surface. It feels natural, looks good in form-fitting clothes, and replaces the weight of your breast. It should last from one to five years.

Permanent breast forms come in a variety of shapes, weights, skin tones, and sizes. It is important that you work with an experienced fitter, particularly the first time you buy one, rather than ordering from a catalog. Working with a good fitter, you should find a form that is just right for you. Once fitted, breast forms should feel comfortable and look natural in your bra and clothes.

A professional fitter will help you determine the weight of the breast form, with the objective of making it correspond to your natural breast weight. This is especially important if your remaining breast is large. Not having the weights balanced may lead to problems with posture as well as neck, back, and shoulder pain. Having the form at the appropriate weight will also help keep your bra from "riding up" on your chest. A large-breasted woman should choose a bra with a large band under the breasts to help carry the weight and reduce pressure on the shoulders.

Women who wear heavier breast forms and an inappropriate bra have an increased risk of developing lymphedema in the affected hand or arm. With too much weight, there's pressure on the bra strap, and that compromises lymphatic drainage across the shoulder. You can avoid this problem by wearing a specially made, lighter form and an appropriate bra. So be sure to try on one of these lighter forms and a good bra at the time of your fitting.

Types of Breast Forms

- **Post-surgical soft form in a camisole**
  A lightweight temporary breast form that fits into a special post-mastectomy camisole. Can be worn immediately after a mastectomy.

- **Non-silicone breast form**
  Another lightweight design made of foam or fiberfill. This type of temporary breast form can be safety-pinned to your undergarments and can be worn immediately after a mastectomy.

- **Weighted silicone form**
  Simulating the shape of a natural breast, this permanent breast form is made of silicone gel. It's weighted to help you maintain normal posture. This form needs to be worn with a bra, generally a custom-fitted post-mastectomy bra.

- **Attachable breast form**
  Convenient for exercising, or when you don't want to wear a bra, this permanent silicone gel form can be attached to the chest with special adhesive strips.

Choosing Comfortable Underwear

Trying to find the right undergarments may take some experimentation. The type of underwear and clothes you choose can help you feel more comfortable, self-confident, and attractive.

After your dressing and drains have been removed, you will probably find that wearing a loose undershirt or camisole made of cotton or silk is more comfortable than wearing your regular bra. Cotton has the advantage of being easy to wash, but you may find silk is especially comfortable if your skin is extra-sensitive to the touch.

Sometimes a garment with some elasticity is preferable to a non-elastic fabric, because the slight pressure on the surgery site feels comforting. You might want to try a sports bra first, because it exerts pressure on both sides, and gives good support to your remaining breast.

But, if you find that a sports bra exerts too much pressure, try a cotton camisole with Lycra. They are available with or without a built-in bra. Or you might want to try a special post-mastectomy camisole with a removable breast form. Soft and loose, this roomy camisole has elastic straps so that you can step into it easily. (That's a big advantage, when you have difficulty lifting your arms.)

Choosing a Comfortable Bra

Sometimes the bra you wore before a mastectomy will still fit afterwards. But immediately after surgery, when your chest is swollen and tender, you may find that it's difficult to try on or fasten any of your bras. If you want to try wearing one of your bras before the swelling goes down, a bra expander might help. The expander, which extends the hook-and-eye section of your bra, can be found in the lingerie section of most department stores.

Even after the swelling has subsided, you may find that your old bras don't fit well any more. Don't hesitate to get refitted for new bras that are the correct size. A professional fitter can measure you and help you find a bra that's comfortable, attractive, and the perfect size for you. If you're being fitted for a permanent breast form, both fittings should be done at the same time. In fact, the key to a well fitting breast form is a well fitting bra. Most permanent breast forms can be worn with any well fitted bra. But, like some women, you may prefer special, post-mastectomy bras with pockets that help to hold the breast form in place.

You want a bra that provides comfort, good support, and is suitable for a permanent breast form. Such bras should have:

- Wide shoulder straps
- Wide band below the cup
- Wide band around your back
- Multiple hooks-and-eyes for fastening

Your First Fitting

The thought of going for a bra and breast form fitting may make you feel uncomfortable. Some women prefer to take an intimate friend to the appointment. A friend can often offer honest feedback as you try out different forms.

How do you find an experienced breast form fitter? Ask your surgeon, nurse, or hospital social worker for a referral. Then call ahead and ask to speak to the fitter. If you find the fitter to be a knowledgeable and caring person, perhaps you'll feel comfortable scheduling an appointment.

Most cities have medical supply stores that carry breast forms. (Look under "medical equipment" in the Yellow Pages, and then for stores that have "breast prostheses.") The atmosphere in these stores, however, may be a bit too clinical for your taste. Many women say they prefer a department store where specially trained saleswomen, in the lingerie department, can help fit them. In some larger communities there may even be specialty stores that cater specifically to women with post-mastectomy needs.

Tips for Fitting

- Wear, or take along, a favorite garment that clearly shows your contours. You and the fitter need to see what you'll look like in your favorite clothes.
- Allow adequate time for your fitting. A trained fitter may need up to one hour to properly fit you.
- When you arrive for your appointment, ask for your fitter by name, so that you can be taken care of discreetly.
- Take as much time as necessary to get the form and bras that you need.

You can expect that your new breast form will feel heavy at first. In time, it will come to feel more natural. Start by wearing the form for about four hours every day, and gradually increase the number of hours that you wear it. Soon you will be able to wear it as long as you need to.

Caring for Your Permanent Breast Form

With proper care, your permanent breast form should last a number of years. The following tips will help make sure it does last:

- Hand-wash the form each day in warm, soapy water. Make sure you use a mild soap such as liquid hand washing or dish washing soap. Never use harsh cleansers or chemicals.
- Rinse the form in warm, clear water.
- Blot it dry with a soft towel. (Never place the form over direct heat.)
- Keep your breast form stored in its original box (in its "cradle") when you're not wearing it.
- Avoid punctures. Be careful that you don't inadvertently puncture the form when you're pinning on jewelry. Here's a tip for cat lovers: keep the form in a closed cradle when you're not wearing it, so it doesn't get scratched by kitty's claws!

Swimming and Sports Breast Forms

Some special breast forms are designed to be worn while swimming and playing sports. You can wear them without a bra and leave them on when you go into a shower, hot tub, or sauna. Unlike permanent breast forms that are held in place by a bra, the sports breast form is held against your chest with a non-irritating adhesive. You first place a special adhesive-backed strip on your chest that can remain in place for as much as a week. Then the breast form attaches to that adhesive strip much like a Velcro fastener. You may remove the form at any time or keep it on twenty-four hours a day.

Will Insurance Pay for Breast Forms?

If you choose to wear a breast form, medical insurance should cover the cost of the fitting and the form. Most insurers will reimburse you for one breast form for each breast every one to two years.

When you purchase a prosthesis, you will likely be asked to pay for it "out-of-pocket," then submit the expense to your insurance company for reimbursement. The cost of breast forms runs from $175 to $450. Ask your surgeon (or any of your doctors) for one prescription for a "breast prosthesis," along with another prescription for "two surgical bras." You should also be reimbursed for one or two bras. Bra prices range from $35 to $45.

Save receipts and copies of the prescription for submission to your insurance company.

Choosing Not to Wear a Breast Form

Finally, there is another choice: wearing no breast form. After a mastectomy, some women choose to go without padding. It is a perfectly valid choice. If you still wish to conceal the fact that you've had a mastectomy, you may find loose-fitting clothes may be all you need. Wearing loose tops over your undershirt and adding more layers, as needed, is an attractive way to conceal your surgery. In colder weather, experiment with vests, sweaters, and jackets. Or you can try draping a beautiful scarf across your chest as one of your layers. In warmer weather, try a vest over a sleeveless shirt or a beautiful scarf over a sleeveless shirt.

If you occasionally wear form-fitting clothes, you might want to consider a breast form. Some women though, feel and look attractive and stylish without padding in form-fitting clothes. As with all aspects of your recovery, do whatever is most comfortable for you.

6

Chemotherapy and Hormonal Therapy

Cancer always seemed like something that happened to someone else. Until now. And, chemotherapy was something that someone else had to go through. But now, you may be considering your own course of chemotherapy. Initially, most women face this prospect with fear and dread. But most women who have gone through it will tell you that it was not as bad as they had expected. Newer medications are effective in minimizing side effects, and many women continue to work during their treatment.

Chemotherapy is often referred to as *adjuvant therapy*, which simply means additional or supporting therapy. It is a systemic therapy—the chemotherapy agents circulate throughout the entire system, or body. How does chemotherapy work? Chemotherapy kills rapidly reproducing cells, cancer cells multiply rapidly, so the chemotherapy agents destroy them. Fast-growing normal cells are also harmed; however, they're capable of repairing themselves.

When Is Chemotherapy Needed?

After a mastectomy, your doctors will be in a better position to judge how your treatment plan should be individualized, based on your surgeon's observation during surgery, a careful analysis of the tissue removed during surgery, and possibly other tests.

Factors that determine whether chemotherapy is needed:

- Your age and general health. The health of your heart and liver are especially important.
- Tumor size.
- Lymph node status. The pathologist will check for the presence of cancer cells in the lymph nodes under the arm on the side of the mastectomy.
- Histology. This refers to microscopic examination of the tumor cells to determine the type of breast cancer and the tumor grade; these indicate how aggressive the cancer is.
- Hormone assay test. This test determines whether the tumor is receptive to the hormones estrogen and progesterone. These hormones stimulate the growth of some breast cancers.
- DNA tests. DNA testing of tumor cells help determine whether the cancer is slow or fast growing.
- Chest x-ray, bone scan, MRI, and CT scans are sometimes used to check for the presence of tumors in the body.

Consultation with the Medical Oncologist

Having chemotherapy is an important decision, so it's essential to have a medical oncologist who is highly qualified.

You want a doctor who will spend time with you, make sure your questions are answered, and put you at ease. Your surgeon will probably recommend a medical oncologist. Make sure the oncologist has the following qualifications:

- Board certification in medical oncology. This means that the doctor has passed rigorous examinations.
- Extensive experience in treatment of breast cancer. You can get this information from your own surgeon, from other breast cancer survivors, or from local advocacy groups.

You may want to take a spouse or friend with you to the appointment with your medical oncologist to listen, take notes, and ask questions. It may be helpful to make a list of any questions you have and take them to your appointment.

Seeking a Second Opinion

During your first visit to a medical oncologist, you need not make a decision about your treatment on the spot. Many women need time to think about what was said during the appointment. It might be helpful to get a second opinion. Your medical oncologist will not feel offended if you seek a second opinion. To the contrary, doctors want you to feel that you are making the best personal choice.

Under what circumstances might a second opinion be helpful? It may be helpful in deciding whether to have chemotherapy if your lymph nodes were negative. Opinions on this matter vary between medical oncologists. And, you may want a second pathology review since there may be a difference in the interpretation of your pathology report. For example, a second opinion may find the tumor to be smaller (or larger) than originally thought. Or, a cancer may be found to be less (or more) aggressive than originally reported. Some larger centers offer a formal second opinion service, in which your pathology slides are sent to expert pathologists for interpretation.

Many times, a second opinion confirms the findings of the first doctor. If you find, however, that the second opinion is substantially different, you may actually need a third opinion.

If you see another doctor, you will need to take copies of your pathology report as well as any other test results from blood work and x-rays. It is wise to have personal copies of all these reports; you may ask the medical oncologist or your surgeon for copies.

How Chemotherapy Is Administered

If you are to receive chemotherapy, you will receive your treatments in your doctor's office or in your hospital's *infusion center*. The session will likely last one to three hours. You'll probably be seated in a comfortable reclining chair. To make yourself more comfortable during treatment, ask for a pillow or light blanket if you need it. For your first treatment, you might feel better if a friend or relative goes along; you may have less anxiety if a loved one stays with you.

Chemotherapy is given on a set schedule. Most commonly, it's administered every twenty-one days, although sometimes it is given weekly or every other week. The total length of treatments is usually three to six months.

Chemotherapy is usually delivered intravenously (IV). Medical personnel usually call this a "drip," since the medication drips from a hanging bottle into your IV. Your oncology nurse or doctor will start an IV in your hand or arm opposite the side of your surgery. You will first receive some hydrating fluids, then powerful anti-nausea medication. When you are well medicated, which may make you feel sleepy, you will be given chemo-therapy. It's important to hold your hand and arm still, so that the IV stays in your vein.

The nurse will let you know when your treatment is completed. Before you leave, make sure you have the name and phone number of the person you may call if you have any questions. If you have any concerns about managing your care at home, don't hesitate to call to get your questions answered. Also make sure that your nurse has given you a written list of your anti-nausea medications and an explanation of when to take them.

Chemotherapy Agents:

Six chemotherapy agents are commonly given as adjuvant therapy for breast cancer. They include:

- *cyclophosphamide* (Cytoxan) (C)
- *methotrexate* (M)
- *5-fluorouracil* (F)
- *adriamycin* (A)
- *paclitaxel* (Taxol) (T)
- *docetaxel* (Taxotere) (T)

These chemotherapy drugs are usually given in combinations, such as CMF, AC, or AC followed by T.

Side Effects of Chemotherapy

Conventional chemotherapy is likely to produce a number of well-known side effects, such as nausea, hair loss, and fatigue.

Some women say they feel like they have a bad flu for about three to five days after each treatment; however many women find that side effects are not as bad as they feared they would be. Many women feel well enough to work during their course of chemotherapy.

Nausea and Vomiting

The nausea associated with chemotherapy has a predictable rhythm. Since you'll be given anti-nausea medications at the time of your treatment, you'll probably feel okay for the first twenty-four hours. The next morning, however, you're likely to begin experiencing nausea, and possibly vomiting. Many women say these side effects peak on the third day. After that, you'll probably start feeling better.

For many women, nausea is the most dreaded result of chemotherapy treatments. However, improved ways of administering chemotherapy and new anti-nausea medications make severe nausea and vomiting the exception, not the rule.

The tips described below will help you cope with side effects.

Drink Fluids

Be sure to drink plenty of hydrating liquids (eight to ten glasses), particularly the day before, the day of, and the three days after chemotherapy. In addition to reducing nausea, fluids flush out the byproducts of chemotherapy and protect your bladder from the chemotherapy toxins.

Take Anti-Nausea Medications

Take these medications on a fixed schedule. Using your medications effectively is key to keeping your nausea under control. Most women need a combination of anti-nausea medications. Medications typically come in three forms: a pill that's taken orally with water, a dissolving pill to be placed under your tongue, or a rectal suppository. Ask your nurse to help you understand exactly how to use the different medications and write down the schedule for you. The most commonly used anti-nausea medications are *Ativan, Compazine, Decadron, Kytril,* and *Zofran.*

If you are vomiting repeatedly, your doctor can prescribe a rectal suppository—most commonly *Compazine*—which usually works well to stop vomiting. Your doctor may also prescribe *Ativan,* an anti-anxiety medication, which may be placed under your tongue.

Vomiting causes dehydration, so take in liquids as soon as possible. If you have gone thirty minutes without vomiting, start hydrating with ice chips. After tolerating ice chips for half an hour, take a tablespoon of water every ten minutes. Thirty minutes later, you should be able to start sipping water. Staying well hydrated helps reduce the cycle of nausea and vomiting.

If these suggestions do not work, then it is important to call your doctor or oncology nurse immediately. Sometimes you may need IV hydration, which requires a visit to your doctor's office, the emergency room, or an infusion center. Severe dehydration is a life-threatening emergency, and it is important to get appropriate medical care as soon as possible.

Eat Small Meals

Eat for comfort. Small, frequent meals every two and a half to three hours are usually preferable to three large meals. When eating seems difficult, choose what appeals to you even if it is not the most "healthy." Carbohydrates seem to work the best, such as potatoes, macaroni and cheese, rice pudding, ice cream, rice, bagels, and toast. Though you may not have much appetite, many women find that eating just a little bit helps calm the stomach.

Try to Relax

Feeling relaxed and comfortable also helps manage nausea. When you're resting, you want a quiet, cool room with dim lighting. Open a window to let in some fresh air. It helps to lie down with a pillow under your head and torso so that they are slightly elevated.

Get Plenty of Rest

Try to get a good night's sleep every night. This may be a challenge, because the treatment itself and medications such as *Decodron*, for nausea, may make it difficult for you to fall asleep. Fatigue will only increase the side effects, so use the sleep medication your doctor prescribes.

Infection

Chemotherapy may lower the count of your *platelets*, white blood cells (WBC), and red blood cells (RBC). Platelets help blood clot. When your platelets are low, you will bruise more easily or you might notice your gums bleeding if you brush your teeth vigorously. White blood cells fight infection, and red blood cells carry oxygen to cells.

In most patients, the blood count plummets to its lowest level some seven to ten days after each treatment. This lowest point is called the *nadir*. Since your WBCs play an important role in fighting infections, when you are at your nadir, your immune system will be weakened and you will be susceptible to viruses and bacteria that can cause infection. Recommendations for fighting infections are listed below.

Seek Antibiotic Treatment

Since the cold virus is very common, you'll be very susceptible to upper respiratory infections. If you have cold symptoms—sneezing, congestion, or runny rose—start taking your temperature three times a day. If you do get a fever, or feel ill, call your medical doctor's office immediately. If your doctor is not available, go to the nearest hospital emergency room. You'll probably be started on a course of antibiotics. Also during the few days of your nadir, avoid crowds and the company of young children, as children tend to get a lot of colds.

Antibiotics will also be prescribed if you should get a bladder infection and/or a vaginal yeast infection. A bladder infection is signaled by an urgent need to urinate frequently and a burning sensation when you do. Two ways to help avoid getting a bladder infection is to be well hydrated to keep the bladder "flushed," and wipe from front to back after each bowel movement to avoid contaminating the urethra.

A yeast infection is indicating by burning or itching and a vaginal discharge. Call your doctor if you have these symptoms.

Monitor Your Blood Count

During chemotherapy, your medical oncologist will carefully monitor your blood count by taking a small sample of your blood with a finger prick. Your body has an amazing capacity to heal, and your blood counts should start rising again after each chemotherapy treatment.

If your WBCs reach their nadir and then remain at a low level, you may need a medication such as *Neupogen* to stimulate the production of white blood cells. Your medical oncologist will be able to tell you whether you can benefit from such a medication.

Washing Hands to Kill Germs
• Wet hands and apply soap.
• Wash the backs of hands as well as palms.
• Rub vigorously to remove bacteria that stick to skin.
• Wash vigorously for twenty seconds.

Wash Your Hands

Studies have shown that the most important way to reduce your risk of catching a cold is simply washing your hands frequently and thoroughly with hot water and soap. Wash your hands as often as possible, especially after going to the bathroom, before eating, and before going to bed at night.

Fatigue

Most people begin to feel tired after their first chemotherapy treatment. This fatigue may continue throughout your treatment. One reason for this is the chemotherapy's effects on red blood cells (RBCs). Consequently, when your red blood cells are at their nadir, they are not delivering oxygen efficiently, and you will feel very tired. This condition is called *chemotherapy-induced anemia*. It will temporarily, but dramatically, add to your fatigue. When you are at your nadir, you may also notice that you have shortness of breath when you exercise or walk up stairs.

There are other reasons you're likely to feel tired. The stress of undergoing surgery and treatment and other side effects are also factors contributing to fatigue.

If your RBCs stay low, and you are very tired, your doctor may recommend a medication, *Procrit*, which stimulates the production of RBCs. Some women find that such medications "work wonders," so be sure to ask your doctor about them.

As previously discussed, walking daily can give you increased energy, so continue walking if possible. At the same time, it's important to conserve energy. Decide what is really important for you to do and what you should let go of. If you work at a full-time job, perhaps you can reduce the number of hours you work during a course of therapy.

Hair Loss

The most obvious physical side effect of chemotherapy is temporary hair thinning or hair loss. Since all hair is made up of fast growing cells, your eyebrows, eyelashes, and pubic hair, as well as the hair on your scalp, will be affected by the chemo-therapy agents.

Most women begin to lose hair from their scalp around the nineteenth day after the first chemotherapy treatment. Once the hair begins to fall out, it usually comes out rapidly—within the following two to three days. For many women, this is an emotionally devastating experience. Many women say that losing their hair was as traumatic to them as losing a breast. But, you can reassure yourself that after treatment your hair will grow back.

While you're coping with the hair loss, you have many resources, including hairpieces, hats, scarves, earrings, and makeup. In fact, a woman can feel confident and attractive during this time.

The key to a natural looking and attractive hairpiece is to have it professionally cut and styled while it's on your head. Consider buying a synthetic wig. They are easy to take care of (they only require shampooing), and many are priced under $300.00. A wig made of human hair may seem desirable, but it's often impractical. The human hair needs constant shampooing, blow-drying, and curling. The cost is nearly four times that of a synthetic wig. Unfortunately, most insurance companies do not cover the cost of hairpieces. If your insurance does, make sure that you get a doctor's prescription for a "cranial prosthesis."

Menopausal Symptoms

Chemotherapy may create a chemically–induced menopause. This occurs in 10 to 50 percent of women younger than forty and in 50 to 94 percent of women over forty.

It occurs because women's ovaries are made up of fast-growing cells, so chemotherapy agents affect them. A woman's period usually stops during treatment. If you're under forty, your period will probably return, but if you're closer to menopause it may not.

Other menopausal symptoms include hot flashes (night sweats) and vaginal dryness. Hot flashes generally lessen over time, although it may take many months. If you're having night sweats, you may wish to review the coping suggestions listed in Chapter 1.

Many women report a lessening of sexual desire during treatment. This is generally temporary. After the completion of chemotherapy, give yourself several months to regain interest in sex. If there's no change, you may wish to speak with your doctor; one possibility is that you have low testosterone levels, as a side effect of the chemotherapy. Also, many counselors are specially trained to talk with you about sexual intimacy, and can suggest steps that lead to enhanced sexual desire.

Memory Loss

Many women notice that while on chemotherapy, they develop problems with short-term memory and concentration. This is often referred to as "chemo brain." But reactions vary. For some women, memory is no problem at all, while others encounter so much memory loss that it actually interferes with daily life. In addition to the chemotherapy itself, memory problems might be aggravated by stress, fatigue, anti-anxiety medications, and the onset of menopause. Any or all of these factors can negatively impact memory. It is important to try to be patient with yourself and compensate for it. When chemotherapy is over, most women who have experienced "chemo brain" find that their memory improves.

Weight Loss

Some women lose weight during chemotherapy. This may occur for several reasons. Immediately after treatments, some women say they have a metallic taste in their mouths. This usually goes away in several days. Meantime, however, it can be challenging to find something to eat or drink that tastes good.

If you experience nausea, you may not feel like eating. Anxiety and depression may also result in loss of appetite.

Some women are pleased to be losing weight; however, it is important to take in enough calories to help your body rebuild tissues damaged during treatment. You might find it helpful to eat several small meals throughout the day. Others find that carbohydrates are easier to consume and often reduce nausea.

Other Possible Side Effects

Some chemotherapy patients report other side effects such as heartburn, gas, diarrhea, and constipation. If you have any of these side effects, do not self-medicate. Call your doctor or nurse.

Some women develop mouth sores that look and feel like cold sores. They occur because the mucous lining of the mouth is made up of fast-growing cells, which are affected by the chemotherapy. You can reduce your risk of mouth sores by avoiding commercial mouthwashes—they are too harsh and drying.

Instead, use a gentler mouthwash by combining one quart of water, one teaspoon of salt, and a teaspoon of baking soda. Use this before going to bed at night and after each meal. Also, your doctor can prescribe a numbing mouthwash or a salve that helps reduce the discomfort.

Hormonal Therapy

Hormonal therapy, also called *endocrine therapy*, is used to prevent the growth or recurrence of breast cancer. To better understand how this therapy works, let's first examine how natural hormones stimulate the growth of some breast cancers.

When cancer cells are analyzed in a pathology lab, pathologists can determine whether the cancer depended on the female hormones, estrogen or progesterone, to grow. If so, the tumors are referred to as *estrogen positive* or *progesterone positive*. In these cases, one of two forms of hormone therapy may be used. One form, the hormonal agent (*tamoxifin*) attaches to cancer cells and prevents them from growing. The second, newer therapeutic agents (*aromatase inhibitors*) block the production of estrogen, essentially "starving" the cancer cells.

Hormonal therapy may be given in place of chemotherapy or in addition to it. Hormonal therapy may replace chemotherapy when the lymph nodes are negative, the tumor is small and slow growing, and the tumor is estrogen positive. Hormonal therapy is routinely given in addition to chemotherapy to women who meet the criteria for "standard" chemotherapy and whose tumors are estrogen positive.

Tamoxifen Therapy

The most commonly used hormonal therapy is *tamoxifen*. More than twenty years of data show tamoxifen has been proven to extend the lifespan of breast cancer patients. An oral medication, tamoxifen (*Nolvadex*) is taken in pill form for five years. The treatment decreases the risk of cancer recurrence in the breast and in other organs. Studies have also shown that women who have had cancer in one breast have a significantly reduced risk of cancer in the other breast when taking tamoxifen.

Side Effects of Tamoxifen

Hormonal therapy is much gentler than chemotherapy, and produces significantly fewer and milder side effects than chemotherapy. Still, tamoxifen may bring on menopausal symptoms such as hot flashes and night sweats. These generally improve over time. Some women report vaginal dryness or vaginal discharge. Other possible side effects include:

- Weight gain
- Slight increase in the risk of blood clots
- Slight increase in the risk of uterine cancer
- Increased depression for those with histories of depression

Other Hormonal Treatments

The newer hormonal treatments, known as aromatase inhibitors, act differently than tamoxifen. They block the production of female hormones. The drug goserelin (*Zoladex*) suppresses estrogen production in premenopausal women. The drugs anastrozole (*Arimidex*), letrozole (*Femara*), and exemestane

(*Aromasin*) block estrogen production in postmenopausal women.

Some women who take aromatase inhibitors have reported joint pain and stiffness. However, when compared to tamoxifen, aromatase inhibitors show a lower incidence of such side effects as endometrial cancer, blood clots, and hot flashes.

Gynecological Care

It's important to see your gynecologist routinely, at least once a year. If you are taking tamoxifen, your gynecologist needs to be particularly attentive to signs of uterine cancer. One warning sign is unexplained vaginal bleeding.

Anyone with a strong family history of breast cancer needs to be monitored for indications of ovarian cancer. A strong family history means that multiple relatives in multiple generations, from either side of your family, have had breast and/or ovarian cancer.

In addition to discussing your family history with your gynecologist, you may also want to meet with a medical geneticist, who is trained to help you and your doctors determine if you are, in fact, at higher risk for ovarian cancer. Although there are no obvious warnings signs of ovarian cancer, a vaginal ultrasound is helpful in screening for both uterine and ovarian cancer, and may be recommended by your gynecologist.

7

Radiation Therapy

Radiation therapy has been used to treat cancer for decades, and advances in modern medicine have made the treatment even more effective. The use of computer tomography (CT) based treatment planning, more sophisticated radiation equipment, and treatment planning computers and software have made it possible to target the treatment area more precisely. As a result, other parts of the body, including the heart and lungs, are spared from significant amounts of radiation. The newer equipment is also skin sparing—the skin is not permanently damaged as it was during treatment in the past.

Approximately 20 to 30 percent of women who undergo mastectomies have radiation treatment. Radiation therapy is not routinely given after surgery, since the intent of the surgery is to remove the cancer. However, radiation is a consideration when a tumor is large or when the cancer cells were found in multiple lymph nodes. The goal of radiation treatment is to kill any remaining cancer in the area of the chest or underarm. Like chemotherapy, radiation is effective in treating cancer because it kills fast-growing cells. As explained in the previous chapter, cancer cells multiply rapidly, making them vulnerable to radiation.

Meeting with Your Radiation Oncologist

In preparation for treatment, you will meet with a radiation oncologist, a physician who is specially trained in treating cancer with radiation therapy. During your first appointment, the radiation oncologist will perform a physical examination and review your medical history. He or she will explain the treatment process and discuss the risks and benefits. This is a good time to bring up any of your concerns. You may wish to ask such questions as:

- Why do you recommend radiation therapy for me?
- What are the common short-term side effects?
- What are the common long-term side effects?
- What can be done to reduce the side effects?
- When I'm having daily treatments, how long will each one last?
- How many weeks will the treatment take?

The Simulation Appointment

Before any treatments are given, you will be scheduled for a simulation appointment. The purpose of the simulation is to determine the precise "treatment field"—the parts of your body where the radiation beam will be aimed.

Once the treatment field is determined, the doctor or radiation therapist will mark your skin, creating a "map" of the area where radiation will be directed. He or she will pinpoint key areas by tattooing tiny permanent blue dots, about the size of a pinhead, on your chest. The therapist then will outline the treatment area with semi-permanent ink. Avoid washing off the ink while bathing.

During the simulation, the radiation specialists will also produce a customized "mold," also referred to as an "immobility device," that will be used to hold your back and arm in exactly the same position during treatments. The device will also help minimize movement. Your simulation appointment will take one to two hours.

Radiation Treatments

Most courses of radiation treatment last about five weeks, with five treatments per week. Radiation therapy is delivered by a machine called a *linear accelerator*. To receive a treatment, a patient lies on a table under the machine.

Before each radiation-treatment session, you will be asked to undress from the waist up and change into a hospital gown. You'll lie on the treatment table with your customized mold under your back and arm. After you are carefully positioned under the machine, the therapist will leave the room and activate the equipment to deliver the radiation beam. The actual treatment may take less than a minute and is painless, much like an x-ray.

You'll receive radiation therapy from two different angles. The therapist will reposition the machine and the second dose of radiation will be delivered.

Once a week, you'll meet with your radiation doctor, who will check your progress. This is another opportunity to ask questions.

Side Effects

Fatigue

During treatment, your body will be working hard to kill cancer cells and to heal from the effects of treatment. One of the

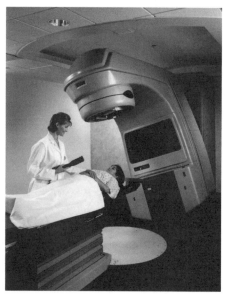

To receive a radiation treatment, the patient is positioned under a linear accelerator as shown above.
Photo courtesy of Varian Medical Systems.

most common side effects of this process is fatigue. Plan to get extra rest. Take a short nap during the day, if you can, and try to get extra sleep at night.

Also continue to take daily walks. As mentioned earlier, a half-hour walk every day during treatment will give you more energy. Also, keep up your exercises, particularly your stretching. If you stop stretching during radiation therapy, you will lose arm flexibility.

A few weeks after treatment ends, you'll probably notice that your energy level has returned to normal.

Skin Changes

Another predictable side effect of radiation is a temporary change in skin color and texture. At first there may be no visible changes, but around the third week of treatment, your skin may show signs of redness and inflammation, similar to a sunburn. The skin may also become dry and feel warm.

To minimize skin discomfort and speed healing, your nurse or doctor will give you instructions about a special skin lotion to use. Use no other lotions on the treatment area. Other lotions may interfere with the delivery of the radiation.

Gently apply only a thin coat of lotion to the whole treatment area, from underarm area to breastbone and from lower bra line up to collarbone. Also, include your shoulder, upper back, and neck. Apply the lotion after each daily treatment, after your bath or shower, and at bedtime, if you desire. Make sure that you do not apply the lotion within two hours before receiving your treatment. For example, if your treatment is at 10:00 A.M., do not apply your lotion after 8:00 A.M.

During radiation therapy, be gentle with the skin over the treated area. Here are some additional suggestions:

- Go without a bra.
- Wear soft, loose, clothing. Never wear tight clothing over the treated area.
- If your skin itches, apply refrigerated cornstarch, patting the area very gently.
- Do not rub, scrub, or scratch the skin.
- When you bathe or shower, use cool water to wash the treated area. Avoid using soap, which can irritate the skin. If you must, use a super fatty soap, such as Basis or unscented Dove.
- Avoid putting anything that is very hot on the area, such as a heating pad. You should never get in a hot tub or take a sauna while you're undergoing treatments.
- Do not apply anything cold, such as an ice pack, to the skin.
- Don't apply powders, creams, perfumes, or body oils that have not been recommended or approved by your nurse or doctor.
- Don't shave your underarm. If you must, use an electric razor.
- Avoid using deodorants or antiperspirants.
- Avoid exposure of the treated skin to the sun. Wear protective clothing and use sunblock lotions recommended by your doctor or nurse.

Other Side Effects

Although it's not common, some women develop a tiny fracture in a rib on the side that was treated. The fracture can cause discomfort, but it is not dangerous and does not require treatment. It heals on its own in a few months.

Some women get a sore throat or dry cough when the treatment area is near the neck or lung. These symptoms usually go away a few weeks after treatment.

8

Breast Reconstruction Options

Each year in the United States, more than 80,000 women of all ages undergo breast reconstruction surgery. Women wishing to have reconstruction surgery have two basic options for reconstruction. The most common choice is *breast implants*. The second choice is *flap surgery*.

Are you undecided about reconstruction? Being unsure is quite common, and the good news is you may determine when the time is right for reconstruction surgery. Nearly half the women having reconstruction elect to have the procedure performed at the same time as the mastectomy. This is commonly referred to as *immediate reconstruction*. Other women choose *delayed reconstruction* which, as the name implies, may be performed months or years later.

Considering Breast Reconstruction

You and your doctors will need to consider several factors as you decide which type of reconstruction is preferable. These factors include your general health, body type, desired appearance, and any post-surgical breast cancer treatment that you've had or will need. Your medical team—surgeon, medical oncologist, radiation oncologist, and plastic surgeon—needs to be involved in planning both your treatment and any reconstruction surgery.

Choosing a Plastic Surgeon

Good communication with your plastic surgeon is essential. Since appearance is a subjective matter, you want your ideas and feelings to be respected. You will want to talk to your surgeon not only before the procedure, but also afterwards. After the operation, it may take many weeks before the bruising and swelling are reduced to the point where you can see what your reconstructed breast really looks like; during this time you will need continued advice and reassurance about the healing process.

The outcome of the surgery depends primarily on the skill and experience of the plastic surgeon. Of course, your surgeon should be board certified which means he or she has had all appropriate training in cosmetic surgery and has passed a rigorous test administered by a board of his or her peers. But perhaps just as important is the doctor's reputation. Look for a surgeon whom other women and medical professionals recommend, based on the surgeon's consistently excellent cosmetic results and low rate of complications.

You'll also want to be sure that the doctor is experienced in performing the type of reconstruction you'll be having. Ask how many years the doctor has been performing reconstructions, and how many procedures he or she has performed. Among other questions you may wish to ask:

- Which procedure does the surgeon recommend for you?
- Where will the scars be, and how will they look?
- Will the reconstruction require more than one operation?

- How long will the reconstruction take?
- How long before the healing is complete?

When you meet with a plastic surgeon, he or she will probably show you before-and-after pictures of other patients whose reconstruction he/she has performed. Remember, you are probably seeing your surgeon's best results. You can also ask to see some results that were not optimal. In addition, you may want to ask the surgeon if you can interview former patients who have undergone the procedure that you are considering. Most doctors are willing to have you contact former patients.

Achieving Symmetry

Plastic surgery is not a perfect art; however, plastic surgeons strive for symmetry, making the two breasts look similar. For women who are having both breasts reconstructed, symmetry is fairly easy to achieve. On the other hand, if you're having one breast reconstructed, achieving symmetry might not be quite as easy. Accordingly, the surgeon might suggest surgery to reduce, lift, or perhaps augment the other breast. Some women are pleased to know these "revisions" are an option; however, if symmetry is less of a concern, you may wish to avoid the additional surgery.

Types of Reconstruction

Breast Implants

A breast implant reconstruction involves the placement of an implant behind the chest muscle (pectoralis), creating a breast mound. Implants may be made of saline solution, which is sterile, salty water, or of silicone—a gel. Or, an implant may be a combination of saline and silicone—the inner pocket is saline, but the outer portion is silicone. Many women believe saline implants feel less like a real breast when compared to silicone implants; they say silicone gel implants have a more natural feel and bounce. Since 1992, silicone implants have had FDA approval for breast reconstruction after mastectomy.

An implant may be a fixed-volume implant, meaning it is already filled to the appropriate size when it's surgically inserted. Or, an implant may be expandable, in which case it serves as a *tissue expander.* The expander, a balloon-like device, is gradually filled over time, stretching the muscle and skin. Ultimately the breast becomes the desired size.

For women with small, rounded, uplifted breasts, fixed-volume implants are the easiest surgical solution—the area under the pectoralis muscle can accommodate a small or moderate-sized implant. However, a woman who wishes to have larger breasts will need a tissue expander. Breast implants may also be the best option when recovery time is a factor. For example, if a woman needs to return to work, she may not have the extra weeks required to recovery from flap surgery.

The operation to insert an implant usually requires one to two hours in the operating room, in addition to the time it takes to perform a mastectomy. Or if a woman chooses to delay the reconstruction, her implants may be inserted during an outpatient surgical procedure.

How Tissue Expanders Work

Once an implant has been surgically placed behind the chest muscle, a woman usually goes to her surgeon's office weekly, over the course of one to three months, for expansion sessions. As saline solution is injected, through an implant valve just below the skin, the implant expands. A typical injection session lasts from five to fifteen minutes. Patients often say that the increased size often causes a temporary, tight, pulling sensation. If you undergo expansion sessions and the process becomes painful, let your doctor know, so that the volume and timing of the next injection can be adjusted. If pain is severe, some filler solution can be removed.

Breast implant placement frequently requires two operations. During the first procedure, the plastic surgeon inserts a temporary expander. After the muscle and breast skin are distended sufficiently, a second operation is performed to replace the temporary expander with a "permanent" implant. Sometimes, however, the expander implant may be converted into a permanent, fixed-volume implant. The surgeon simply removes the valve used for the expansion process.

Why can some women keep the temporary expander when others need a replacement or permanent implant? First, understand that there are many choices for implants—different shapes, sizes, and textures. The surgeon chooses the one he

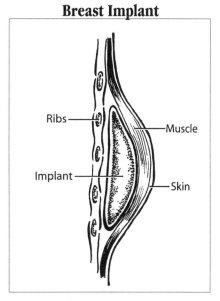

Breast Implant

Ribs

Muscle

Implant

Skin

or she believes will produce the best cosmetic result. For some women, the expander is cosmetically attractive and may be left in place. Other women will achieve a better result with a different permanent implant.

Advantages of Implants

The main advantage of breast implants over other kinds of reconstruction is a shorter recovery time. The recovery time is similar to that of a woman having a mastectomy without reconstruction.

Disadvantages of Implants

Implants do not last indefinitely. Even without complications, they may have to be replaced after about twelve years. Why? The outer shell may break down, causing leakage. If this occurs, a surgeon might have to remove the implant and replace it; this may be done in an outpatient surgical procedure.

Sometimes, a hard fibrous scar tissue, a *capsular contracture*, forms around the implant. In some cases, the capsular contracture becomes tight, the implant hardens, and the breast appears deformed. A surgeon can resolve this problem by performing a *surgical capsulectomy*, in which the thickened capsule and implant are removed and the implant is repositioned, replaced, or removed.

Another disadvantage to implants that use tissue expanders is the months of asymmetry during the expansion process. As the process begins, the reconstructed breast is smaller than the other breast; then it becomes larger as the implant is expanded for several weeks before it is converted to the permanent implant.

Finally, some women object to the idea of having a foreign substance in their bodies. These women may prefer another reconstruction option such as flap reconstruction.

Flap Reconstruction

The alternative to a breast implant is a *flap reconstruction*. Surgeons can reconstruct one or both breasts using a flap that consists of a woman's own skin, fat, and muscle. Many women prefer flap reconstruction because their own tissue produces a breast that is more natural.

What criteria determine whether a woman is a candidate for a flap procedure? In addition to good general health, a woman needs adequate fat tissue in the abdomen (for an abdominal flap). Women who smoke, who are obese, or who have diabetes are not ideal candidates for flap surgery.

Flap reconstruction may also be an option when implants are not possible. For example, if a woman has had radiation therapy and her skin has become "inelastic," the use of an implant may not be possible.

The most common flap reconstruction is a *pedicle flap* procedure, in which the base of the flap stays attached to the body and is "swung around" to form the breast. By keeping the flap attached to the body, the flap's blood supply is undisturbed, assuring that the flap tissue stays alive and healthy. The two types of pedicle flaps are the *TRAM flap* and the *latissimus dorsi flap*.

The second basic type of flap procedure is known as a *free flap*. This procedure involves a more extensive operation in which the donor flap is totally removed from the body and then used to form the new breast. This procedure requires microscopic surgery to connect blood vessels and arteries.

All flap reconstructions are major surgeries, requiring four to six hours in the operating room. Accordingly, recovery time is longer than with implant surgery.

TRAM Flap

The TRAM (*transverse rectus abdominis muscle*) flap is the most common type of flap reconstruction. For this procedure, the donor flap is taken from the lower abdomen and pulled upward to the chest to form a breast.

For this operation, the surgeon creates the flap, leaving the base of it attached to a portion of the vertical abdominal muscle. The flap is elevated and transferred to the chest wall area through a tunnel the surgeon creates under the upper abdominal skin. The upper part of the flap is sutured into position in the breast area, and the lower portion of the flap is positioned, folded under, and contoured to form a breast mound.

During the operation, the patient is moved to an upright position on the operating table so that the breasts can be checked for symmetry. By having the patient in a sitting position, the surgeon may better assess the natural drape of the breasts. Once the breasts are symmetrical, the flap is carefully stitched in place.

A secondary benefit to a TRAM flap procedure is a flatter stomach or "tummy tuck." This is the result of the surgeon removing the abdominal flap and tightening the remaining muscles of the donor area, restoring strength to the abdominal wall.

During a TRAM operation, one or two breasts may be reconstructed. However, this type of operation can be done only once. If a

TRAM Flap

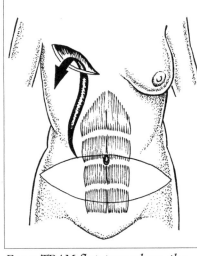

For a TRAM flap procedure, the flap is taken from the abdomen. The pedicle flap stays attached to the abdominal muscle under and to the inner part of the breast.

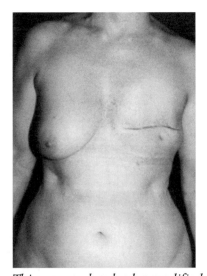

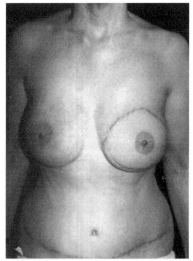

This woman has had a modified radical mastectomy.

Photos courtesy of Loren Eskenazi, M.D.

The same woman is shown here after her breast was reconstructed with a delayed TRAM flap procedure.

woman undergoes a TRAM flap operation for one breast, and the need arises for reconstruction to the other breast, a different reconstructive procedure will be required.

About six to eight weeks after surgery, the postoperative swelling will have resolved. Then, both you and the plastic surgeon can see the size and contour of your new breast. Frequently a surgeon will recommend further minor surgery to improve the contours of your reconstructed breast or your stomach. In some cases, the surgeon may suggest a simple "touch-up" with an outpatient liposuction procedure, in which excess fat is sucked from the breast and/or stomach.

Latissimus Dorsi Flap

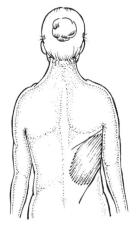 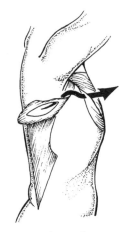

For a latissimus dorsi flap procedure, the flap is taken from the back, just below the shoulder blade.

The latissimus dorsi flap is pulled under the skin around to the chest, and a breast mound is formed.

Latissimus Dorsi Flap

For this procedure, the flap is made up of part of the latissimus dorsi muscle, the large flat muscle on the back, immediately below the shoulder blade. As with all pedicle flaps, this flap stays attached at the base and is pulled around and under the arm to form the breast.

During the operation, the surgeon creates the flap, rotates it, and passes it through a tunnel under the skin in the underarm. The donor site is closed with sutures. The flap is adjusted for the most aesthetic appearance and sutured to the front of the chest; the latissimus dorsi muscle is stitched to the pectoralis major muscle, and the skin is stitched to the chest skin.

When doing a flap reconstruction, the plastic surgeon has an opportunity to create a very natural-looking breast, one that has a natural drape. Size may vary from small to quite ample. If the tissue from donor area in the back doesn't provide enough bulk, the surgeon may also use an implant to create a larger breast mound.

Free Flap Reconstruction

As the name suggests, the free flap procedure involves "freeing" or totally removing a flap of skin and tissue from the body to form a new breast. The free flap procedure is a more complex operation, since microsurgery is required to reconnect veins and arteries once the flap is in place.

Because the flap is totally removed in the free flap procedure, the source of the donor flap need not be limited to the abdomen or the back. The free flaps may be taken from the abdomen, back, buttocks, hip, or thigh.

The surgeon first makes an incision at the mastectomy site, making a space for the flap. After the flap is transferred to the breast region, the blood vessels of the abdominal flap are sutured into the blood vessels in the armpit area. During this final, critical part of the procedure, the surgeon uses an operating microscope.

When the blood vessels have been connected and checked, the muscle of the flap is firmly sutured to the underlying chest wall. The overlying skin and fatty tissue are shaped to form a breast.

In deciding whether to choose a free flap rather than a pedicle flap procedure, there are a number of considerations. One is the experience of your surgeon. Not all reconstructive surgeons have performed the free flap procedure, and great skill is required to suture the minuscule veins and arteries. When an experienced surgeon is available, however, it's reasonable to consider the free flap procedure.

Advantages of Flap Reconstruction

Each type of flap reconstruction carries certain risks and benefits. It is important to discuss the options in detail with your surgeon. The main advantage to flap surgery: it produces a more natural breast, since it's made from one's own tissue. Also, flap reconstruction produces a breast that is truly permanent, unlike implants that may need to be replaced.

When a free flap is used, there is less trauma to the body than with a pedicle flap, because the surgeon doesn't need to cut tissues between the chest and the donor site in order to "tunnel under" with the flap.

Disadvantages of Flap Reconstruction

Scars

There is always a scar at the donor site where the flap was lifted away. Scars can be quite large. A TRAM flap procedure leaves a "bikini scar" that runs horizontally from one hip to the other. The latissimus dorsi procedure leaves a long scar on the back. A free flap procedure leaves a scar in the thigh, buttock, or other donor area.

With the latissimus dorsi procedure, if a large amount of skin and fat are removed from the back to create a large breast, healing time may be extended. The resulting scar might be unattractive, and the back area from which the flap was taken could appear flatter then the opposite side of the back. In addition, there may be a slight bulge under a woman's arm where the flap was tunneled. This bulge will shrink in time as the muscle atrophies, but it will not completely disappear. Some women report that it is difficult for them to keep their shoulder erect on the side of the muscle transfer. Physical therapy can help but may not totally eliminate this problem.

The flap reconstruction is a major surgery. Consequently, pain associated with flap procedures is more intense than with an implant surgery, and the recovery time is longer.

Potential Healing Problems

Because any kind of flap reconstruction is major surgery, there are several potential complications. About one in ten patients experience some healing problems, resulting in an area of skin loss or an area of flap loss. Sometimes healing is delayed because of insufficient blood supply, but rarely is the entire flap lost. Sometimes a clump of fat dies and it forms a hard lump. Usually this lump can be removed surgically or with liposuction. Sometimes such fat lumps soften without removal, though the softening may take six to eight months.

Other potential complications include the formation of a seroma, a pocket of lymph fluid under the skin or a *hematoma*, a pocket of blood under the skin. If you see any signs of these problems, call your surgeon right away.

You should also call your doctor immediately if you experience pain, swelling, or a sensation of warmth in the calf of your leg. These symptoms could mean the formation of a blood clot. Do not rub or massage your legs. Doing so could dislodge the clot. If you can't reach your surgeon immediately, go to an emergency room.

Creating a Nipple and Areola

Most women heal from breast reconstruction surgery after several months. At that time, the plastic surgeon can reconstruct the nipple and areola. This is usually performed as an outpatient procedure. Most commonly, the surgeon creates the nipple using a small flap of skin from the center of the reconstructed breast itself; the skin is "spiraled" and molded to form a nipple. As an alternative, a nipple and areola may also be reconstructed with a skin graft from the abdomen or inner thigh. The surgeon may then tattoo both the nipple and areola for a good color match. Surgeons often create the areola with only a tattoo. The tattoo procedure is quick, painless, and simple; however, the tattoo may fade in time.

When it comes time for nipple reconstruction, some women hesitate about having yet another surgical procedure. Although these feelings are understandable, keep in mind that you won't feel pain during the procedure. Of course a local anesthetic will be used, but also your reconstructed breast will still be somewhat numb. A nipple and areola significantly enhance the final outcome of the reconstruction.

One of the most commonly asked questions is, "Will my new nipple and areola have any sensation?" Whether one has a breast implant or a reconstructed breast, unfortunately, the answer to this question is "no."

Does Insurance Pay for Reconstruction?

Yes, insurance pays for breast reconstruction surgery. Since the passage of the Women's Health and Cancer Rights Act of 1998, insurance companies have been required to pay for breast reconstruction for women who want it.

9

Recovery from Reconstruction Surgery

We spoke in the first chapter about how surprised most women are to find that having a mastectomy was not as difficult physically as they had thought it would be. However, that is not exactly the case with recovering from a flap reconstruction surgery. And not to mince words, most women report that recovering from flap surgery is a slow, painful process.

Women report the most discomfort with the TRAM flap procedure. Some compare it to an abdominal hysterectomy or a Cesarean section. The pain in the chest will be somewhat less since nerves were cut during surgery, but abdominal nerves remain intact, so it is common to feel more pain in the abdomen. Despite the discomfort, women typically say that it was worth it.

Your Hospital Stay

After surgery, you will be in the hospital for four to six days. You will be sleepy most of this time since you'll be receiving pain medication. Most women do not feel up to visitors, except for family and close friends.

You will have several drains. Usually, you'll have one at each end of the abdominal incision and two drains in the breast—one near the underarm and one near the mid-chest. These drains will remain in place when you go home. While you have the drains, you cannot take a bath or shower, so the nurse's aide or nurse will help you wash.

Pain Management

For the first few days, when the pain is the most intense, you will have a pain management device called a patient-controlled analgesia unit (PAC). The PAC unit is connected to your intravenous line (IV), and you can press a button to administer the pain-relieving medication as needed. The machine is set so that there's no chance you can get an overdose. After three to four days, you will make the transition from the PAC unit to an oral narcotic pain medication.

Narcotic pain medication slows down your whole body, and that includes your bowels. You will be given stool softener in the hospital, and the nurses will want you to have a bowel movement before you go home. You might need an enema before you're discharged.

Getting Out of Bed the First Time

On the second day, the nurses will remove your catheter and you'll need to get out of bed to go to the bathroom. Even though the nurses will help you, getting out of bed will likely be painful. Why? Because if you had a TRAM flap operation, some of your stomach muscles were cut, and we use our abdominal muscles to pull ourselves up. Before standing up, give yourself a dose of pain medication and brace your abdomen with a pillow if your flap was taken from your abdomen.

When the nurses first help you up from the bed, you will not be able to stand up straight. In fact, it may take several weeks before you are able to stand completely straight, depending on the tightness of your abdomen.

Moving around Your Room

Standing and moving may be so uncomfortable at first that you might be tempted to stay in bed. This is not a good idea. You need to walk to prevent complications such as blood clots in the legs, a condition referred to as *deep vein thrombosis*. A clot could travel to the lung, causing a *pulmonary embolism*; a potentially life-threatening complication, an embolism obstructs blood flow in the lung. You will also wear support hose to further enhance the blood flow to and from the legs, reducing the chance of blood clots.

Recovery at Home

For most women, the first few weeks at home are a challenging time physically and emotionally. You will need someone with you full time, from one to three weeks, to help you with all aspects of your care. This includes intimate care such as help with bathing and going to the toilet.

Plan to have someone prepare meals and do housework for at least three weeks. If you have children who need care, you may want them to stay with a close relative or friends. If you prefer that they stay home with you, older children need to know that they will have to help, and younger ones will need child care. You simply won't be able to pick up a child or do other housekeeping

Items to Have Ready at Home

- Hospital bed (may be rented for two or three weeks)
- Recliner chair
- A firm-seated chair with arm rests
- Elevated toilet seat
- Portable commode
- Many extra pillows
- A bell for the bedside (to call for assistance)
- Plastic bench for shower or bathtub
- Hand-held shower head for bath or sink (to help you wash your hair)

tasks. This in itself can be frustrating if you're not used to being dependent on others.

Pain Management at Home

Each woman has a different tolerance for pain. After leaving the hospital, some women are comfortable taking only over-the-counter pain medication, while others need prescription pain medication for many weeks. Your doctor will prescribe a pain medication, usually the same one you took in the hospital, for you to have filled when you go home. Review the pain management suggestions on page 4.

Sleeping

At first, you will probably have some problems getting comfortable and sleeping through the night. If you have a partner, you may want to consider sleeping alone for a while, for your comfort as well as your partner's.

Your prescribed pain medication will help you fall asleep, so be sure to take it at bedtime. Have a night stand prepared with things that you need—a lamp, a glass of water with a straw in it, and your pain pills. You might want a bell on a side table, just in case you need assistance. If it's a long way from your bedroom to the bathroom, you may want to have a portable commode at your bedside.

Sleep in the flexed position so that you don't put a strain on your abdomen. If you have had a TRAM flap reconstruction, sleep on your back, elevated at a forty-five degree angle. If you do not have a hospital bed or recliner chair that can be adjusted, ask someone to place several large pillows behind your back to elevate your body. Place more pillows under your affected arm to lift it higher than your heart. You will also need to elevate your knees by adjusting the bed or having someone insert pillows under your knees. When your abdomen feels comfortable, you are in a good position.

If you have had the latissimus dorsi reconstruction, the most comfortable sleeping position is lying on your unaffected side rather than on your back. Place several pillows under your torso and under your affected arm.

Getting Out of Bed

To make getting out of bed easier, first turn on your affected side, assuming a fetal position, then use your unaffected arm to push off the bed. Position yourself on the edge of the bed, with your legs about twelve inches apart. Use a pillow to brace your abdomen, and then use your leg muscles and your unaffected arm to lift yourself.

Each day practice standing up straight. This will help stretch your tight abdomen. In about two to three weeks, you should be able to rise to a normal standing position.

Getting up from bed is not a problem for women who have had the back flap (latissimus dorsi) procedure, since the belly muscle has not been cut.

Getting Out of a Chair

The most comfortable chair during recovery is one with a hard seat and sturdy arms. (A chair with a soft seat-cushion puts tension on your abdomen when you sit.) When you're sitting, if your legs don't reach the floor, place a cushion under your feet, so you're putting less strain on your abdomen. Before getting up from the chair, position yourself near the edge, legs twelve inches apart, and use your legs and unaffected arm to push yourself up. Brace your abdomen with a pillow as you rise.

For additional comfort, you will probably want an elevated toilet seat, so you don't strain your abdomen when you sit or stand.

Grooming and Dressing

For about two weeks, you'll need help when you bathe and wash your hair. As long as the drains and stitches are in place, you will need to take sponge baths rather than immersing yourself in a tub or taking a shower. You'll be able to handle most other parts of your grooming routine—brushing your teeth, washing your face, and combing your hair.

Choose comfortable, loose clothing that's easy to put on, such as soft, loose shirts or robes that open in the front. When putting on a shirt, place your affected arm in the sleeve first. Choose pants with a very loose waistband since your waistline will be temporarily swollen.

What to Eat and Drink

You may eat whatever appeals to you, and it is always important to drink plenty of hydrating liquids, such as plain water and herbal (non-caffeinated) teas. To enhance wound healing, it is important to eat protein, fruits, and vegetables; also take a daily multi-vitamin. Because your abdominal area is tight, you may feel full after eating only a small amount of food. If so, try eating small, frequent meals. The tightness in your abdomen will loosen in time.

Getting more fiber in your diet is important since you are likely to experience constipation as a result of prescription pain medication and inactivity.

Resuming Normal Activities

Gradually, you'll recover mobility and strength, and you'll be able to resume normal activities. Early on, do remember the importance of walking—it helps keep the blood flowing. Walk from room to room and even up and down stairs. Walking on stairs does not put pressure on your abdomen. As soon as you feel up to it, you may go outside to walk. You can begin gently using your affected arm. In fact, on the second day at home, you may begin the stretching exercises described in chapter 2.

You'll probably find that you can gradually get back to normal activities, such as light housework, cooking, and shopping about three to five weeks after surgery. But assume that it will take at least eight weeks before your energy level feels normal.

More rigorous activities will have to come later. It probably will be three to six months before you'll be able to engage in sports.

Taking Care of Your Incision

If you have had delayed reconstruction and you had a mastectomy some time ago, you probably remember taking care of your incision. However, if you've had immediate reconstruction, this will be new to you.

As mentioned in a previous chapter, the main thing to watch for is signs of infection—redness, swelling, warmth, pain around the incision, or excess drainage. If you notice a soaking stain on your underclothes, call the surgeon's office immediately.

You probably won't have a dressing over your incision, so wear something soft, comfortable, and washable next to your skin. Whatever you're wearing is likely to get stained from the normal drainage.

Taking Care of Your Drains

The drains in your reconstructed breast and in the donor site help the healing process by draining blood and lymph fluid which normally collect after surgery. As the drains fill, they need to be emptied according to directions you received from the hospital nurse.

You should notice less drainage each day. Note, too, how the color changes from reddish pink to straw color, the color of lymph fluid. If you notice that no fluids are being collected, there may be a clog in the drain. Use the "milking" technique, described in Chapter 1.

How Will Your New Breast Look?

When you first see your new breast, it won't look like those you saw in the "before and after" pictures your surgeon showed you. You may feel disappointed and discouraged. Some women even question whether they made the right choice. With your reconstructed breast, underarm, and tummy still swollen from the surgery, none of the proportions look right. Your reconstructed breast may look too big, and perhaps your tummy is not as flat as you'd hoped it would be. The bruising may be extensive. And, without a nipple and areola, your breast may look even more odd to you.

Rest assured, the swelling will slowly subside, and the bruising will disappear. Over the weeks the colors will change from a dark blue to purple to a light yellow. If you had a TRAM procedure, your surgeon had to reconstruct a "new" belly button; this, too, may look different from your natural one (it may also be located in a slightly different part of your tummy). And it will also look more natural once the swelling subsides. After a pedicle flap operation, there's also some fullness in the inner portion of the reconstructed breast. But in two or three months, that too will subside.

So remember when you take that first look in the mirror, you *will* look and feel dramatically better in six to eight weeks. Remember those "after pictures" that your surgeon showed you—those women recovered. Remind yourself: this condition is temporary. In time, most women who have undergone reconstructive surgery are very happy with their appearance.

Noting Sensory Changes

After breast reconstruction, you are encouraged to touch your incision, your breast, your underarm, and your tummy to experience the different sensations. You won't hurt yourself by doing this. You'll find out which areas have lost feeling and which areas are extremely sensitive to touch.

As your incision heals, a scar will form. Like your mastectomy site, a healing ridge will form. In time the ridge will soften. While the scar is healing, it may itch. Massaging a mild unscented lotion into the scar will make it feel more comfortable.

Post-Operative Visits

The first post-operative visit after reconstruction surgery is similar to the follow-up visit after mastectomy. Some of the drains may be removed, but others may be kept in place. Drains are usually removed when the drainage is less than 24 ccs (less than one ounce) during a 24-hour period. Removable stitches are taken out in five to ten days after surgery. Others may stay in place longer.

If you've had immediate reconstruction, this may be the time your surgeon will review the pathology report with you. The report will contain results of lab tests conducted on the cancer cells, and possibly lymph nodes, removed during your operation. Following this initial visit, you will meet once a week with your plastic surgeon about three or four more times. After that, your visits will probably be less frequent, depending on how you are healing.

Your First Shower or Bath

The morning after your surgeon removes all your drains and all your stitches, you can take a shower (not a bath—that comes later). To reduce the risk of infection, you should shower every day and wash your incision with mild soap and water. Using the pads of your fingers or a washcloth, make circular motions, working your way from one end of the incision to the other. The incision will probably feel numb. Some women are hesitant to wash the incision, fearing that it will "open up." This simply won't happen. Pat the incision dry, always using a clean towel. Make sure that the incision is completely dry before you put on clothing. Use your clean fingers to gently massage a topical antibiotic ointment, one recommended by your surgeon, into all your incisions including your navel.

Usually, you can take a full bath after all your drains have been removed and all your incisions are well healed. If you want to take a soaking bath, ask your surgeon first.

Driving

The guidelines for driving after a mastectomy apply after reconstruction surgery. If you are no longer taking any narcotics for pain, you may begin driving when you feel ready. For some women that can be in as soon as three weeks after discharge from the hospital.

Going Back To Work

Some women are ready to go back to work in six weeks. Discuss this with your doctors. Always, the priority is to take care of yourself so that you maximize the healing. If what you do on the job is not conducive to healing, your return to work should be postponed.

10

Understanding Lymphedema

Lymphedema is chronic swelling caused by an accumulation of *lymph fluid* in the tissues, which may result when lymph nodes are removed. In the case of breast cancer surgery, several lymph nodes are often removed from the underarm area. As a result, patients are at risk for lymphedema occurring in the affected arm, hand, or the fingers.

You are at risk for lymphedema if you:

- have had multiple auxiliary lymph nodes removed from under the arm.
- have had radiation therapy in your underarm area.
- are diabetic.
- get very little exercise.

How the Lymph System Works

To better understand lymphedema, let's first examine the body's lymph system. The system, made up of lymph vessels, capillaries, and nodes, moves lymph fluid throughout our bodies. The lymph system has two main functions. First, as part of your immune system lymph fluid carries white blood cells, which fight infection. Second, the lymph system helps remove excess fluids (swelling) that collect at an injury or surgery site. Such swelling, also called *edema,* gradually subsides as the lymph drainage system carries away the excess fluid.

How Lymphedema Develops

When lymph nodes are removed, your lymphatic system is easily "overloaded." The lymph system is no longer as capable of carrying away the extra fluid in the tissues of your affected hand and arm. That is why you are susceptible to the chronic swelling that characterizes lymphedema. Lymphedema may occur soon after surgery, or it can occur anytime over the course of your life. Some women have developed lymphedema as long as twenty years after surgery.

Why Lymph Nodes Are Removed

During breast cancer surgery, a surgeon may remove several lymph nodes from the underarm area, called the *axilla,* to test them for the presence of cancer cells. If cancer cells are found, it's an indication that the cancer has spread outside the breast. In performing *axillary lymph node sampling,* a surgeon typically removes between seven and fourteen lymph nodes, out of a total of approximately thirty-five in the area. (The body has about 800 lymph nodes.)

But whether or not cancer cells are found in the lymph nodes, removal of the axillary nodes creates a risk for developing lymphedema. The more lymph nodes are removed, the higher the risk of developing lymphedema.

Fortunately, a new procedure to test lymph nodes, the *sentinel node biopsy,* involves removing only one or two lymph nodes. This surgical advancement places women at minimal risk.

Stages of Lymphedema

The first sign of lymphedema is often subtle. Maybe there is a slight swelling in one part of your affected hand or arm. At first, the swelling may only develop on the wrist or a single finger. If you receive treatment for lymphedema in the early stages, you will be able to prevent it from getting worse. There are three categories or "grades" of lymphedema.

Grade I

The earliest stage, grade I or *acute lymphedema*, is also referred to as *pitting edema*. You can tell if it is present by pressing on a swollen area with your finger. If you see an indentation or "pit," you may have an early stage lymphedema. The swelling should promptly go down if you elevate your arm. Acute lymphedema generally responds to prompt and proper treatment. If, however, you do not receive proper treatment, the lymphedema may progress to grade II lymphedema, usually after three to six months.

Grade II

In grade II, swelling on the affected side becomes more obvious. The tissue feels "spongy" and is *non-pitting*, which means when the skin is pressed with a finger it does not pit. The skin bounces back. With grade II lymphedema, the skin also hardens as fibrous tissue develops, a condition called *fibrosis*. The hardened tissue further blocks lymph flow, which makes the lymphedema worse.

Grade III

At this stage, the swelling becomes extensive. The skin and underlying tissue become hard or fibrous. If lymphedema goes untreated, there's an added risk of an infection, *cellulitis*, which may form as a result of the stagnant excess fluid collecting in the tissues; this fluid is full of protein, which is "food" for bacteria.

Cellulitis: A Medical Emergency

If you have cellulitis, you may have a rash, and your skin will be slightly swollen and warm to the touch. If cellulitis progresses, you may develop one or several red lines running up your arm. Then, in the short span of a few hours, a large area or the whole arm may become very red, swollen, hot, and quite painful. These infection symptoms indicate full-blown cellulitis. At this point you may also feel tired and unwell, and you may even have a fever.

As soon as you see any symptoms of cellulitis, seek medical attention immediately. You will need appropriate antibiotic therapy, which usually starts with oral antibiotics, followed by IV therapy if the condition worsens. Without treatment, cellulitis can lead to septic shock (blood poisoning) and eventual death.

A small wound, particularly if it's properly treated, typically does not develop into cellulitis. But, if any cut or sore becomes infected and you let it go, there is a real danger of this infection turning into cellulitis. If cellulitis is developing, you can usually better detect the signs by examining your skin in natural daylight.

Treatment for Lymphedema

Lymphedema Therapists

Unfortunately, most medical doctors lack specialized training to treat lymphedema. However, hundreds of certified lymphedema therapists are available in the United States and Canada. Some nurses, physical and occupational therapists, and licensed massage therapists, as well as a small number of medical doctors, are trained in lymphedema therapy. Contact the National Lymphedema Network, listed in the Resources section in this book, for suggestions on finding a trained therapist near you.

Lymphedema Therapy

Any swelling that persists for more than three days needs to be evaluated even if the swelling goes down after elevating your arm. Ideally, you should start treatment within two weeks of noticing any persistent swelling.

A woman undergoing lymphedema treatment should have several treatments a week for four to eight weeks or until swelling subsides. Treatment sessions last about an hour. The most effective treatment will include the following steps:

- Education. Since the risk of lymphedema lasts a lifetime, it's important to know as much about it as possible.
- Antibiotic therapy. Before treatment can actually begin, you must be free of infection. The lymphedema therapist will evaluate you for any signs or symptoms of infection and will work with a doctor to prescribe appropriate antibiotic therapy (usually penicillin).
- Cleaning and lubricating the skin.

- Manual Lymph Drainage (MLD). With this special massage technique, the therapist uses gentle pressure to move the fluid back into the vascular system and reduce swelling.
- Bandaging and wrapping the hand and arm. After MLD is performed, the therapist wraps the hand and arm with special bandages (not Ace or elastic type bandages). The greatest pressure is on the hand; pressure is decreased on the higher parts of the arm. The bandage stays on until the next treatment.
- Breathing and muscle-building exercises. After the bandages are applied, the therapist will have you perform several breathing and muscle contraction exercises that increase lymphatic flow and drainage.
- Compression sleeve. At the end of the course of treatments, you will be fitted with a compression sleeve. The sleeve replaces the bandages and wrapping. This sleeve is worn during the day to maintain the benefits of treatment and to prevent or slow the accumulation of fluid.
- Regular follow-up. Routine follow-up is important. Each year, you may need additional treatment.

Preventing Lymphedema

Many of the things you do every day can affect your risk for lymphedema. By modifying how you dress, work, exercise, and travel, you may be able to reduce your risk to a minimum. Pay special attention to the following lifestyle factors.

Avoid Tight Clothing and Jewelry

It's important to avoid wearing tight rings, watches, or bracelets that could constrict lymph flow. You also need to avoid carrying a heavy purse, handbag, or luggage with a strap that goes over your affected shoulder. And avoid any garments, such as those with tight wrist bands, that constrict blood flow to the arm.

If you wear a breast form or prosthesis that weighs heavily on your bra straps, you will need to be refitted with a lighter form. The constriction of vessels in your affected shoulder can lead to or worsen lymphedema.

Avoid Repetitive Stress Injuries

Working nonstop at any task that involves your affected hand and arm, especially if you do it for several days in a row, may lead to lymphedema. Most people are aware that working improperly at the computer is one cause of repetitive stress injury, but there are other causes as well. Tasks such as gardening, knitting, drawing, and painting may also lead to stress injuries.

To avoid these injuries, take a short break every twenty minutes and stretch your upper body, especially your hands and arms. Also, do regular, moderate exercises to strengthen your hands and arms.

Exercise

Regular, moderate exercise reduces your risk for lymphedema and infections by stimulating lymphatic flow and improving circulation. Water aerobics and swimming are excellent forms of exercise for preventing lymphedema. The water acts like a natural compression garment for your arm, and it also keeps you cool, so you don't risk overheating. Being overheated may lead to dehydration, which increases the risk of lymphedema.

Be Cautious with Vigorous Exercise

If you enjoy more strenuous activities such as weight training with heavy weights, long distance bike riding, tennis, cross country skiing, or basketball, you need to take some specific precautions to avoid lymphedema. Why? When you exercise strenuously, the muscles in your upper body fill with blood. This can overload your lymphatic system. Similarly, injury to a muscle may cause fluid to collect.

If you notice swelling when you perform an exercise or sport, you need to consider modifying or giving it up. But the following tips may enable you to continue exercising safely:

- Don't exercise to the point that you are sore. When muscles hurt, it means you have injured muscles.
- Drink plenty of water and don't push yourself on hot days.
- Pace yourself. Take breaks at least every twenty minutes to stop, breathe, and stretch.
- If you develop swelling during an exercise session, stop immediately.
- Wear a "lymphedema sleeve" on the affected arm. This specially designed sleeve is like support hose for your arm, exerting the most pressure near your wrist. Purchase a correctly designed sleeve. Don't make it yourself. Wear it for activities such as golf, tennis, biking, or strength training.
- Avoid very hot showers or baths, saunas, hot tubs, or steam rooms especially after a vigorous workout.

Plan for Air Travel

Air travel, and preparing for it, increases your risk for lymphedema. This happens for several reasons. Often, you're busy before taking a trip—cleaning your home, washing, ironing, and packing. The activity may overload the lymphatic system. The day of the flight, you may be carrying a heavy suitcase; you may reach and strain if you place your baggage on an overhead bin.

During the flight you may become dehydrated since air in the plane is very dry. And you stay seated for many hours, impeding blood flow. You may be hot and thirsty when the plane lands. That's when you may notice that your hand or arm is swollen.

You can avoid at least some of these problems if you take the following measures:

- In the days before your trip, pace yourself; and don't overuse your affected arm.
- Do not carry heavy baggage on your affected side. Get help if you need to place heavy items in the overhead compartment.
- Stay well hydrated. Drink a lot of fluids and avoid alcohol or caffeinated drinks, which are dehydrating.
- Reserve a seat where your affected arm is not near the aisle, where it might be bumped and injured by a passenger or beverage cart.
- Every hour, move about the cabin and perform five "arm pump" exercises.
- Wear a compression sleeve for the entire flight.

Preventing Injury and Infection

Since the lymph system is part of your immune system, you are at greater risk of getting infections from even small cuts or wounds. And any untreated infection can lead to lymphedema. Preventing injury and infection is especially important for women who have diabetes; diabetics have a higher risk of infections since their healing ability is often impaired.

Preventing Wound Infection

If you get a scrape, scratch, or cut on your affected side, you must treat the wound appropriately, even if the wound seems quite small. To prevent getting cuts and scratches it's a good idea to wear protective gloves and clothing for tasks that might lead to injury, such as housework, home maintenance, yard work, gardening, and baking.

If you do suffer a wound, here are steps you should take to prevent infection:

- Vigorously wash the wound with soap and warm water for at least 20 seconds, twice a day.
- Apply a topical antibiotic to the wound. Prescription Bactroban (mupirocin calcium cream 2 percent) is the best topical antibiotic.
- Cover the wound with a Band-Aid or sterile gauze dressing, and keep it dry.
- Check the wound twice a day for any signs of infection, which include redness, swelling, warmth, pus, and increased pain.

If you take these preventive measures and still see signs of infection, you'll need oral antibiotics. If you cannot reach your doctor, go to an emergency room.

Some doctors will give you prescription antibiotics in advance if you plan to travel or if you live far away from a pharmacy. This can be very helpful if you enjoy camping or plan to travel internationally. Also, ask your doctor about topical and oral antibiotics that you can carry with you.

Prevent Fingernail Infections

The hand on your affected side requires some special attention, particularly in the area around your fingernails, which may become infected if you get a hangnail. Give yourself gentle manicures by gently pushing back your cuticles. Don't cut the cuticles, since they protect your nail from infection. Use your own manicuring tools and don't share them. Make a habit of cleaning them with rubbing alcohol.

If you enjoy having your nails done professionally, take your own manicuring tools to the manicurist. Unfortunately, many nail salons do not sterilize their instruments, so it's essential to take your own.

Avoid applying artificial nails. Toxic chemicals are used to apply them, and the chemicals tend to ruin the natural nail. This can be a source of fungal infection.

Prevent Insect Bites

Some women develop large welts when bitten by insects. Such injuries may lead to lymphedema. The best measure is prevention. Wear long-sleeved shirts and apply insect repellent liberally. If you do get bitten, here's what to do:

- Take an antihistamine (such as Benadryl), which will help reduce swelling.
- Take an anti-inflammatory drug (such as Advil).
- Apply topical cortisone cream to reduce inflammation.
- Apply an ice compress, twenty minutes on and ten minutes off.

With treatment, any welt caused by an insect bite should resolve in an hour or so. If it doesn't, you should call your doctor.

Prevent Skin Irritation

Your skin acts as a barrier that keeps bacteria and viruses from entering your body. But even this infection barrier may be impaired if your skin is dry and cracked. To keep your skin pliant, always use mild soaps, such as Cetaphil, Basis, and unscented Dove, particularly on your affected hand and arm. After you bathe, vigorously but gently rub your skin with a towel to remove dry and dead skin. Then apply a lotion. Eucerine is especially good because it lowers the pH (increasing the acidity) of your skin. When the pH is lower, it inhibits bacteria growth.

When you shave under your arm, you may accidentally cut the skin, particularly if that area is numb to the touch. The best policy is to use an electric razor rather than a straight-edge razor.

It's also important to prevent sunburn. Wear protective clothing or use a generous amount of sunscreen when you're going to be outdoors for any length of time.

11

Follow-up Care

Y ou've made it through a breast cancer diagnosis. You've made it through a mastectomy, and perhaps chemotherapy or radiation. Now, in many respects, you are resuming a "normal life." Still, in the back of your mind is the scary thought that breast cancer can recur. Virtually every woman who has had a mastectomy copes with these thoughts.

Hopefully you will be reassured by the fact that you'll still maintain contact with your doctors through follow-up care. If no health problems arise, doctors usually like to see patients every three or four months for five years. After five years, most doctors like to see a patient twice a year.

Before an Appointment

Before doctor appointments, note any subtle changes in your body that you have noticed since the last visit. Some women find that it's helpful to keep a "symptom journal." If you notice a new symptom, describe it and note the date it started. If the symptom causes discomfort, grade the severity of the discomfort, using a scale from 1 to 10, with 1 being mild discomfort and 10 being severe pain. With such a record, you'll see a pattern of any symptoms.

Certainly, you would want to contact your medical oncologist immediately if you're having any pain or persistent symptom that lasts for more than two weeks. A symptom that comes and goes away is *not* a sign of cancer recurrence.

Follow-Up Visits to Your Surgeon

Your surgeon is the best doctor to give you a thorough breast examination. He or she will be watchful of any signs of cancer at the mastectomy scar, the most common site of local recurrence. Your doctor will also carefully check your unaffected breast. The surgeon will be looking for:

- A lump or thickening on the mastectomy scar, or a lump on the reconstructive breast
- A rash or black-and-blue mark that does not go away
- An enlarged, non-tender lymph node in the armpit or above the collar bone

Once a year, your doctor will want a mammogram of your unaffected breast. If you had breast reconstruction with either an implant or with your own tissue, you will not need a mammogram of your reconstructed breast.

Follow-Up Visits to Your Oncologist

During your regularly scheduled visit, your medical oncologist will take a careful history, perform a physical exam, and when appropriate, order tests. Your medical oncologist will be checking you for signs of metastatic disease, that is, any indications that cancer may be found in other parts of your body. The most common kinds of metastatic disease, in order of prevalence, are bone, lung, liver, and brain metastasis.

The oncologist needs your help to detect symptoms that may be of concern. If you report certain symptoms, the doctor may then decide to have tests done. Since you and the doctor are working hand in hand to monitor your health, it will be helpful to be aware of symptoms of metastatic disease so that you can report them immediately.

Symptoms of Bone Metastasis

A localized pain that hurts continually may be sign of a tumor growing within the bone. The pain may not necessarily feel like it is coming from the bone, but it is constant—it usually remains at night and it does not improve with time.

If you report this kind of pain, the medical oncologist will usually order an x-ray and bone scan tests. A bone scan is a diagnostic test in which a small amount of radioactive substance is injected into the bloodstream. By tracing the radioactive substance, a scanner can detect any areas of increased blood circulation in the bone, indicating the presence of cancer.

Symptoms of Lung Metastasis

Usually a tumor in the lung does not cause pain. However, if a tumor takes up space in a major airway, it might cause breathing problems such as shortness of breath and a constant, dry cough. These symptoms typically get worse. A medical oncologist may use chest x-rays to make a diagnosis.

Symptoms of Liver Metastasis

Symptoms of a liver metastasis result from a tumor that is taking up space in the liver and impeding its function. Symptoms may be subtle at first, but may include unexplained and worsening fatigue, weight loss, loss of appetite, and nausea. Cancer in the liver may also cause discomfort in the right abdomen, above where the liver is located.

The first test a doctor is likely to order is a simple blood test that will reveal whether liver enzymes are elevated. If so, an oncologist will probably request a CT scan or ultrasound scan of the liver. A CT scan, a computer-aided x-ray, shows three-dimensional images of the liver. Ultrasound testing uses a high-frequency sound wave to check the liver.

Symptoms of Brain Metastasis

A symptom of a brain tumor is a constant headache. But, of course, many women get tension headaches that have nothing whatever to do with a tumor. The difference is that a headache associated with brain metastasis typically begins in the morning, before one gets out of bed, but then improves as the day goes on. This is different from a tension headache, which usually starts during the day and then gradually gets worse. Be sure to tell your doctor about any recurring headaches and try to describe them as thoroughly as possible.

There are other possible symptoms. Sometimes drowsiness, nausea, or both accompany these headaches. Some patients have seizures. Other symptoms may be similar to those having a stroke—an inability to walk, weakness in parts of the body, or vision problems.

To make an accurate diagnosis, oncologists rely on a CT scan or an MRI, a diagnostic test that uses a powerful magnet and radio waves to show the number of blood vessels in tissue. Since cancers have more blood vessels than healthy tissue, brain tumors show up as distinct images in a CT scan or MRI.

Can Recurrence Be Detected Early?

Some medical oncologists perform blood tests to detect *antigens*, substances which some breast cancer tumors shed into the blood stream. Also known as *tumor markers*, these substances may signal the presence of cancer in the body. If tumor marker levels decrease after chemotherapy or hormonal treatment, it indicates a good response to treatment. If tumor marker levels increase, it may be a sign of resistance to treatment or a recurrence. Three tumor marker tests commonly used to detect breast cancer are Cancer Antigen 15-3 (CA 15-3), and Cancer Antigen 27.29 (CA 27.29), and Carcinoembryonic Antigen (CEA).

Note however that these tests are not sensitive enough to detect very early recurrences since a tumor must be large enough to release detectable tumor markers. Also, these tests may yield false positives, indicating a positive or abnormal result when, in fact, no abnormal condition exists. It's recommended that all three tests listed here be used to enhance accuracy.

Performing Monthly Breast Self-Examinations

You are encouraged to do a breast self-examination (BSE) every month. Although many mastectomy patients initially find it scary to examine themselves, in time they find it easier. In fact, by learning how to effectively examine yourself, you may feel more in control and less fearful. You will be examining the side of the mastectomy, your unaffected breast, and your affected underarm. Breast self-examination will allow you to detect any changes that may be of concern, such as a lump, a visual change, arm swelling, or infection.

During this visual exam, notice whether you have any of the following changes and tell your surgeon about them:

- Persistent rash or a black and blue area on your scar, chest and/or breast
- Persistent itchy rash on your nipple or areola
- Nipple discharge that is spontaneous and persistent
- A change in the size or shape of your breast, such as a dimple
- Any lump in your breast, chest, scar, or underarm area

Ask your doctor or nurse to show you how to do a BSE, or check with your local hospital to find out if there is a nurse who can teach you BSE.

Appendix

Types of Breast Cancers

Ductal Carcinoma In-Situ (DCIS): earliest stage of breast cancer in which "cancer like" cells are confined to the milk ducts.

Invasive Ductal Carcinoma: cancer that has invaded the tissues outside the milk ducts. The most common form of breast cancer, it comprises 80 percent of breast cancers.

Lobular Carcinoma In Situ (LCIS): abnormal cells are found in the lobules, where milk is produced. Cells are not malignant, but are a "marker" for cancer.

Invasive Lobular Carcinoma (ILC): cancer that has broken through lobule membranes. ILC makes up 10 percent of breast cancers.

Less Common Types of Breast Cancer

Inflammatory Breast Cancer: an aggressive cancer that spreads to the lymphatics of the skin and often throughout the body. Makes up 1 percent of cases.

Tubular Cancer: ductal cancer that has "tube-like" projections. Makes up 1 to 2 percent of cases. Less aggressive.

Medullary Carcinoma: invasive ductal cancer. Tumors resembles brain tissue. Makes up 6 percent of cases. Favorable diagnosis.

Papillary Carcinoma: invasive ductal cancer, comprising 1 to 2 percent of cases, has finger-like projections. Favorable diagnosis.

Paget's Disease: a rare cancer found in the nipple and areola. Makes up 3 percent of cases. Highly curable.

Mucinous Carcinoma: invasive ductal cancer that produces mucus. Found in 3 percent of cases.

Breast Cancer Stages

Breast Cancer is generally divided into five stages. A woman's prognosis, or chance for disease-free survival, is strongly linked with the stage at which the cancer is diagnosed.

Stage 0: Ductal Carcinoma In Situ (DCIS) or Lobular Carinoma in Situ (LCIS) any size.

Stage I: Invasive cancer that measures two centimeters in diameter (approximately ¾ inch) or less and is confined to the breast.

Stage II: An invasive tumor that measures larger than two centimeters, but not larger than five centimeters in diameter, and/or has spread to the lymph nodes under the arm.

Stage IIIA: An invasive tumor measuring larger than five centimeters in diameter and/or has spread to the axillary lymph nodes.

Stage IIIB: An invasive breast cancer of any size that has spread to the skin or chestwall.

Stage IV: Invasive cancer, regardless of size that has spread to distant sites such as bones, lungs, liver, or brain.

Don't try to determine the stage of your own breast cancer. Staging is a complex process. Women may frighten themselves needlessly by trying to stage their own cancer. For example, a woman with a large ductal carcinoma in-situ (DCIS), measuring 6 cm, may think that her stage is 3A—when in fact, the actual stage would be 0, and her lifetime risk of survival is 99 percent with appropriate treatment.

Resources

Breast Cancer Action

55 New Montgomery St., Suite 624
San Francisco, California 94105
1-415-243-9301

An activist and advocacy organization of breast cancer
survivors and their supporters; its purpose is to increase the
awareness of breast cancer among those in government, the
scientific community, private industry, and the media. The
organization publishes a newsletter.

The Susan G. Komen Breast Cancer Foundation

5005 LBJ Freeway
Suite 250
Dallas, TX 75244
Phone: 972-855-600
www.komen.org
www.breastcancerinfo.com

A nonprofit organization with a network of volunteers in local
chapters throughout the United States, this foundation

organizes the *Race for the Cure* events in cities across the United States. Its mission is to eradicate breast cancer as a life-threatening disease by advancing research, education, screening, and treatment.

National Coalition for Cancer Survivorship (NCCS)

1010 Wayne Avenue
Suite 770
Silver Spring, MD 20910-5600
Phone: 301-650-9127 or 877 NCCS-YES (877-622-7937)
www.cansearch.org

Founded in 1986 by and for people with cancer and those who care for them, NCCS is a patient-led advocacy organization working on behalf of people with all types of cancer and their families. Its mission is to ensure quality cancer care for all Americans by leading and strengthening the survivorship movement, empowering cancer survivors, and advocating for policy issues that affect cancer survivors' quality of life.

The Breast Cancer Fund (TBCF)

2107 O'Farrell Street
San Francisco, CA 94115
Phone: 415-346-8223
www.breastcancerfund.org

TBCF (or "The Fund") is a nonprofit organization formed in 1992 to innovate and accelerate the response to the breast cancer crisis. The mission of The Fund is to end breast cancer and to make sure the best medical care, support services, and information are available to all women.

National Alliance of Breast Cancer Organizations (NABCO)

9 East 37th Street, 10th Floor
New York, NY 10016
Phone: 888-80-NABCO, or 888-806-2226
www.nabco.org

NABCO is a nonprofit organization offering information and educational resources on breast cancer. NABCO provides information to medical professionals, patients and their families. It advocates beneficial regulatory change and legislation.

Celebrating Life Foundation (CLF)

P.O. Box 224076
Dallas, TX 75222-4076
Phone: 800-207-0992
www.celebratinglife.org

This nonprofit organization is devoted to educating the African-American community and women of color about the risk of breast cancer. CLF encourages advancements in the early detection and treatment among these women, and works for the improvement of survival rates.

American Cancer Society (ACS)

15999 Clifton Rd NE
Atlanta, GA 30329-4251

Phone: 800-ACS-2345 (800-227-2345)

www.cancer.org

A national, non-profit organization with local chapters that provides education, emotional and practical support programs. The ACS "Reach for Recovery" program provides one-to-one emotional support and information by trained volunteers who are breast cancer survivors. "Look Good. Feel Better." is a free workshop for women undergoing treatment for cancer. The workshop covers using turbans, scarves, wigs, and makeup. The ACS web site offers news and health information about the nature of breast cancer and its causes, risk factors, and treatment. The site also features message boards and chat rooms.

Cancer Care, Inc.

275 7th Ave.

New York, NY 10001

Phone: 800-813-4673

www.cancercare.org

A nonprofit organization since 1994, Cancer Care offers emotional support, information, and practical help to people with all types of cancer and their loved ones. All services are free. Oncology social workers are available for phone consultations in which they provide emotional counseling and support. Cancer Care also offers education seminars, teleconferences, and referrals to other services.

Y-Me National Breast Cancer Organization

212 W. Van Buren, Suite 500
Chicago, IL 60607
Phone: 312-986-8338
24-hour Y-ME National Breast Cancer Hotlines:
800-221-2141 English
800-986-9505 Spanish
www.Y-ME.org

In addition to its advocacy role, Y-Me provides information, peer support, and referral. Y-Me has chapters throughout the country that offer support groups, and its web site is available in Spanish as well as English. Callers can talk with trained volunteers who are breast cancer survivors.

AMC Cancer Research Center & Foundation

1600 Pierce Street
Denver, CO 80214
Phone: 303-233-6501
800-321-1557
800-535-3777 Cancer Information and Counseling Line
www.amc.org

This not-for-profit research institute is dedicated to the prevention of cancer and other chronic diseases. AMC conducts cancer research in the areas of causation and prevention. Its other areas of research are nutrition (for the prevention of disease), health communications, behavioral research, and community studies.

The National Lymphedema Network (NLN)

Latham Square, 1611 Telegraph Avenue, Suite 1111
Oakland, CA 94612-2138
Tel: 510-208-3200
Fax: 510-208-3110
Infoline: 1-800-541-3259
www.lymphnet.org

The NLN provides education for the prevention and treatment of lymphedema. Its hotline offers support, information, and referrals for treatment of lymphedema. The NLN publishes a quarterly newsletter.

The Cancer Information Service (CIS)

National Institutes of Health
Bethesda, MD 20892-2580
Phone: 301-496-4000
1-800-4-CANCER (800-422-6237)
www.cancernet.nci.nih.gov

The National Cancer Institute is part of the National Institutes of Health and is the federal government's principal agency for cancer research and control. The CIS offers free written material and information about treatment, support services, medical facilities, second opinion centers, and clinical trials. Trained information specialists answer cancer-related questions.

OncoLink

The University of Pennsylvania Medical Center
3400 Spruce Street— 2 Donner
Philadelphia, PA 19104
www.oncolink.upenn.edu/disease/breast

Maintained by the University of Pennsylvania, OncoLink's mission is to help cancer patients, families, health-care professionals, and the general public receive accurate cancer-related information at no charge. OncoLink offers comprehensive information about specific types of cancer, updates on cancer treatments, and news about research advances. The information (updated every day) is provided at various levels, from introductory to in-depth.

The U.S. National Library of Medicine

8600 Rockville Pike
Bethesda, MD 20894
www.nlm.nih.gov
MEDLINEplus www.nlm.nih.gov/medlineplus

Produced by the National Library of Medicine, this site indexes articles from more than 3,500 medical journals. The service is aimed primarily at scientists and health professionals; however, MEDLINEplus is written for consumers.

Glossary

A

adjuvant therapy: Treatment added to increase the effectiveness of primary therapy—such as chemotherapy, hormonal therapy, and radiation therapy. Usually done after surgery to prevent or delay local or systemic recurrence.

aneuploid: Containing abnormal amounts of DNA; aneuploid tumors are fast growing tumors.

areola: Area of pigmentation around the nipple.

asymmetrical: Having opposite parts that do not match, as when one breast is larger than another.

axilla: Armpit.

axillary lymph nodes: Lymph nodes that are located in the armpit area. Breast cancer cells can travel to the axillary lymph nodes. One of these—called a sentinel node—or a number of them may be removed to test for the presence of cancer cells.

axillary lymph nodes sampling: The surgical removal of some of the lymph nodes found in the armpit region.

B

bilateral: Involving both sides, as in a bilateral mastectomy.

blood count: Blood test to measure the number of red blood cells, white blood cells, and platelets.

bone scan: Test to determine the presence of cancer in the bones.

bone marrow: The soft inner part of large bones that produces red blood cells, white blood cells, and platelets.

BRCA1 and BRCA2: Mutated genes associated with hereditary breast and ovarian cancer. May be inherited from father's or mother's side of the family. About 10 percent of breast cancers are inherited.

breast implant: A pouch filled with saline solution or silicone gel that is surgically implanted beneath the muscle and skin of the chest to form a reconstructed breast.

breast reconstruction: The surgical creation of the breast contour, nipple, and areola. Performed by a plastic surgeon.

breast self-examination (BSE): The examination of the breast, chest, and lymph nodes by a woman herself.

C

cancer: A general term for more than one hundred diseases characterized by the abnormal and uncontrolled growth of cells. Also called malignancy.

carcinogen: Substance that can cause cancer.

carcinoma: Cancers that arise from the skin, the lining of internal organs, and glands. Breast carcinoma arises from the milk-producing glands and/or ducts.

CAT scan: A study that creates three-dimensional images of organs and structures inside the body. Used to detect the presence of cancer in the major organs in the body.

cell: The smallest structural unit of living tissue that can survive and reproduce on its own.

cellulitis: Infection of soft tissue. The tissue becomes red, hot, swollen, and painful.

chemotherapy: Cancer treatment using cytotoxic (cell killing) drugs. Chemotherapy is administered when there is the risk that cancer cells have spread.

clavicle: Collarbone.

clinical breast examination: An examination of the breast, chest, and lymph nodes performed by a health care provider. The examination consists of a visual and a touch (palpation) examination.

cytotoxic: Causing the death of cells. The term usually refers to drugs used in chemotherapy.

D

DCIS (ductal carcinoma in situ): The earliest stage of breast cancer in which abnormal cells remain in the ducts and have not broken out or invaded (infiltrated) the surrounding tissue. DCIS is also referred to as intra-ductal cancer.

differentiated: Clearly defined. Well differentiated tumors closely resemble normal cells and are slow growing.

diploid: Containing normal amounts of DNA; diploid tumors are slow growing.

DNA (deoxyribonucleic acid): The genetic material contained in the nucleus of the cell. The DNA of cancer cells is analyzed to see whether they have the normal amount of DNA (diploid) or an abnormal amount (aneuploid).

donor site: The part of the body from which tissue is taken and transferred to the breast for reconstruction. The abdomen or upper back are the most common donor sites for breast reconstruction.

drain: A suction device that is inserted during surgery to drain fluids that accumulate after surgery.

ducts: The channels in the breast that carry milk to the nipple.

E

edema: Swelling caused by a collection of fluid in the soft tissue.

erb B2: Another name for the Her-2 neu oncogene. See Her-2 neu.

estrogen: Female sex hormones produced by the ovaries, adrenal glands, placenta, and fat. There are three types: estriol, estradiol, and estrone.

estrogen receptor: Protein found on some cells to which estrogen molecules will attach. If a breast cancer tumor tests positive for estrogen receptors, it is sensitive to estrogen.

F

fat necrosis: Area of dead fat that may develop after surgery or trauma. May appear as a lump or thickened tissue.

flap: A portion of muscle, fat, and skin and its blood supply that is moved from one part of the body to the chest to reconstruct a breast.

G

gene: The basic unit of heredity. Each gene occupies a certain location on a chromosome, a linear thread in the nucleus of a cell.

genetic: Relating to genes or inherited characteristics.

grading: Classification of cancers according to the appearance of cancer cells under the microscope. Low-grade cancer grows more slowly than high-grade cancer.

H

hematoma: A mass of blood that can form in a wound after surgery or after a trauma.

Her-2 neu (or erb B2): Name of an oncogene which when over expressed, leads to more cell growth.

hormone: A chemical substance produced by a gland or a number of glands. There are many kinds of hormones, which act like chemical messengers. They enter the bloodstream and cause effects in other tissues.

hormone assay test: Diagnostic test to determine whether a breast cancer's growth is influenced by hormones (estrogen or progesterone) and can be treated with hormonal therapy.

hot flashes: Sensation of heat and/or flushing that occurs suddenly. May be associated with menopause or may be a side effect of some medications, such as chemotherapy and hormonal therapy.

hysterectomy: a surgical procedure in which the uterus is removed.

I

immune system: The body's system for promoting healing and killing viruses, bacteria, and cancer cells.

infiltrating cancer: Breast cancer that has broken out of the milk ducts and/or lobules and infiltrated surrounding tissue. Infiltrating does not imply that the cancer is fast growing or that it has spread outside the breast. Infiltrating has the same meaning as invasive.

inflammatory breast cancer: A particularly aggressive form of breast cancer that is usually treated with chemotherapy first, and then with a mastectomy and radiation therapy.

inspection: Visual examination.

L

Latissimus dorsi flap: A section of muscle, skin, and fat that is taken from the upper back muscle and used to form a reconstructed breast.

LCIS (lobular carcinoma in situ): Atypical lobular cells. The presence of LCIS indicates a higher risk for developing either invasive lobular or invasive ductal cancer in either breast.

linear accelerator: The machine most commonly used to deliver radiation therapy.

lobule: The part of the breast that produces and stores milk.

local recurrence: Reappearance of the cancer at the site of the original tumor.

local treatment: Treatment of breast cancer by surgery and radiation therapy.

lumpectomy: A surgical procedure that removes the cancer and a rim of healthy tissue around the tumor. This breast conservation procedure is usually followed by six to seven weeks of radiation therapy to the breast.

lymphedema: The chronic swelling of the hand and/or arm. This condition is a possible lifelong complication from removing the lymph nodes in the axilla or treating axillary lymph nodes with radiation therapy.

lymph nodes: Small, bean-shaped glands found throughout the body that help eliminate bacteria, viruses, and cancer cells.

M

malignant: Cancerous.

mastectomy: The surgical removal of the breast. A modified radical mastectomy removes the breast and some of the lymph nodes under the arm. A simple mastectomy removes only the breast.

metastasis: The spread of breast cancer cells to another organ, such as the bones, lungs, liver, or brain.

micrometastasis: Microscopic and as yet undetectable but presumed spread of cancerous cells to other organs.

modified radical mastectomy: Surgical removal of the breast and some axillary lymph nodes. The chest wall muscle is not removed.

MRI (magnetic resonance imaging): A diagnostic test that uses a powerful magnet and radio waves to detect cancer in different organs in the body.

mutation: An alteration in the structure of a gene.

N

nadir: The lowest point in a patient's blood count, usually seven to ten days after a chemotherapy treatment.

necrosis: Death of tissue.

negative lymph nodes: Lymph nodes that are free of cancer cells.

neoadjuvant therapy: Chemotherapy or hormonal therapy given before surgery.

nucleus: The central body of a cell that is the essential agent for cell growth, metabolism, reproduction and transmission of the characteristic of a cell.

O

oncologist: A doctor who specializes in the treatment of cancer. A radiation oncologist specializes in the treatment of cancer with radiation therapy; a medical oncologist specializes in treatment with medication; and a surgical oncologist specializes in treatment with surgery.

oncology: The study of cancer.

oncology nurse: A nurse who specializes in the care and recovery of persons with cancer. She or he is a good resource for symptom management, educational material, and information on emotional support.

P

palpation: Examination by touch.

pathologist: A doctor who specializes in examining tissue under a microscope and diagnosing disease.

pathology report: A pathologist's report of the analysis and tests performed on tissue removed in surgery.

pectoralis major and minor: The major muscles that lie under the breast and over the rib cage.

plastic surgeon: A doctor who specializes in surgically creating a breast contour, nipple, and areola.

platelets: Cells in the blood that help the body stop bleeding.

poorly differentiated: refers to cancer cells which look very different from normal cells and are fast growing.

progesterone: A female hormone. See hormone assay test.

prosthesis: An artificial substitute for an absent part of the body, such as a breast prosthesis (form) or a cranial prosthesis (hair piece or wig).

ptosis: Drooping.

R

radiation oncologist: A doctor who specializes in treating cancer patients with radiation therapy.

radical mastectomy: Surgical procedure that removes the breast, underlying muscles, and axillary lymph nodes. Sometimes referred to as a Halsted Radical. This operation is no longer performed.

radiologist: A doctor who interprets imaging studies such as mammography, MIR, bone scan, and CT scan, to diagnose disease.

recurrence: Return of the cancer after the initial treatment.

red blood cells (RBC): These cells (erythrocytes) give blood its color. Their purpose is to carry oxygen from the lungs throughout the body.

retraction: A drawing-in of the nipple or the skin of breast, which can be a sign of breast cancer.

S

S-phase fraction: A measurement of how many cells are dividing at a given time; if the S-phase is low, this indicates a slow-growing tumor; if it is high, this indicates a fast-growing tumor.

saline: A sterile, saltwater solution. Some breast implants are made of saline.

sentinel node: The first lymph node that drains from the tumor; therefore, the first node in which spreading cancer cells are likely to show up.

sentinel node biopsy: A surgical procedure that removes the sentinel node for examination under a microscope. If the sentinel node is free of cancer, the other axillary nodes do not need to be removed and examined, so that pain, nerve damage, and the risk of lymphedema are minimized.

silicone gel: Silicone produced in a semi-solid state used as a filling in breast implants; similar in consistency to normal breast tissue.

simple or total mastectomy: The surgical removal of the breast. The lymph nodes and pectoralis muscles are not removed.

sporatic breast cancer: The type of breast cancer that is not inherited. Ninety percent of breast cancers are sporatic.

symmetrical: Balanced. One side matches the other.

systemic treatment: Treatment of the whole body, such as chemotherapy and/or hormonal therapy.

T

tamoxifen (Nolvadex): Oral medication commonly used as hormonal therapy for estrogen receptor positive tumors. Has been used and studied for twenty years, and has been demonstrated to reduce the rate of recurrence.

tissue expander: An adjustable implant that is inflated with saltwater to stretch the chest muscle and skin after a mastectomy.

toxic: Poisonous.

TRAM flap breast reconstruction: A breast reconstruction technique that uses a section of muscle, skin, and fat from the abdomen to form a breast.

trauma: Wound or injury.

tumor: Abnormal mass of tissue.

U

Ultrasound (sonogram): A test that uses high-frequency sound waves to generate images of internal organs or tumors. An ultrasound can determine whether a lump is a benign, fluid-filled cyst or whether it is solid.

W

White blood cells (WBC): These cells (leukocytes) are part of the body's defense against infection.

Index

Indole-3 carbinol, 34
infection, 6, 74–76
  fingernail, 124
  cellulitis, 117
  prevention, 123–125
  signs of, 12
  wound, 123
infusion center, 70
insect bites
  prevention, 124, 125
insufficient blood supply, 101
insulin, 34
insurance
  breast forms, 65–66
  reconstruction, 102
  wigs, 77
intercourse, 52
intimacy, 50–51
intravenous (IV), 70, 104

J

Japanese diet, 32, 33
job, 14, 15, 113

L

lack of sensation, 13
latissimus dorsi flap, 95, 98, 99
libido
  loss of, 54
lifting, 4
linear accelerator, 85
liposuction, 97
liver metastasis, 129
lotion, 86, 87
lung metastasis
  symptoms of, 128

lymph fluid
  see also lymphedema
  excess, 19, 25, 114
lymph node, 11, 68
  axillary, 114
  enlarged, 127
  removal, 4, 14, 115
  system, 114, 115
  tenderness, 127
lymphedema, 25, 29, 61, 114–125
  acute, 116
  development, 115
  prevention, 119–122
  stages, 116, 117
  therapists, 118
  therapy, 118, 119
  treatment, 118, 119

M

magnetic resonance imaging (MRI), 68, 130
mammogram, 127
manual lymph drainage (MLD), 119
massage, 50
mate
  talking to your, 49, 50
meats, 36
medical oncologist, 68, 69, 89, 90
medications
  anti-nausea, 72, 73
  for depression, 54–56
  over-the-counter (OTC), 5
memory loss, 78, 79
menopausal symptoms, 78
mental health professional, 54
metastatic disease, 127

Index

About the Author

Rosalind Benedet, R.N., M.S.N., N.P., is the director of the Breast Cancer Recovery Program at the California Pacific Medical Center's Breast Health Center in San Francisco. A certified nurse practitioner in women's health, Ms. Benedet received her nursing degree and her master's in nursing science at the Massachusetts General Hospital Institute of Health Professionals in Boston. She is a native of San Francisco.

Ms. Benedet is also the author of *Understanding Lumpectomy—a Treatment Guide for Breast Cancer* (Addicus Books, 2003).

Also from Addicus Books...

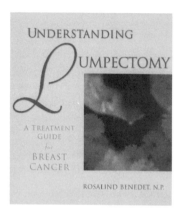

Understanding Lumpectomy
A Guide to Breast Cancer Treatment

Rosalind Benedet, R.N., Mark Rounsaville, M.D.

Research now shows that lumpectomy and radiation therapy is as effective as mastectomy for some invasive breast cancers. In this unique book, oncology nurse Rosalind Benedet guides readers through the surgical procedure as well as follow-up treatment which may include radiation or chemotherapy. 164 pages.

$14.95

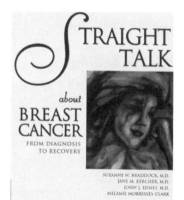

Straight Talk About Breast Cancer: From Diagnosis to Recovery

Suzanne Braddock, M.D., John Edney, M.D., Jane Kercher, M.D.
Melanie Morrissey Clark

After recovering from a double mastectomy and chemotherapy, Suzanne Braddock, M.D. wanted to write a book that answers the pressing questions women have after a diagnosis. She achieved that goal with this book, which is now used by hospitals, clinics, and state health departments across the country. Eight pages of reconstruction photos. 172 pages.

$14.95

Other Consumer Health Titles
from Addicus Books
Visit our online catalog at www.AddicusBooks.com

A Simple Guide to Thyroid Disorders *$14.95*

Straight Talk About Breast Cancer From Diagnosis to Recovery. *$14.95*

The Stroke Recovery Book—A Guide for Patients and Families *$14.95*

The Surgery Handbook—A Guide to Understanding Your Operation. . . . *$14.95*

Understanding Lumpectomy: A Treatment Guide for Breast Cancer *$14.95*

Understanding Parkinson's Disease: A Self-Help Guide *$14.95*

Organizations, associations, corporations, hospitals, and other groups may qualify for special discounts when ordering more than 24 copies. For more information, please contact the Special Sales Department at Addicus Books. Phone (402) 330-7493. Email: info@AddicusBooks.com

Please send:

_____copies of _____
                                                    (Title of book)

      at $_____each   TOTAL   _____

      Nebr. residents add 5.5% sales tax   _____

      Shipping/Handling
         $4.00 for first book.
         $1.00 for each additional book.   _____

         TOTAL ENCLOSED: _____

Name _____

Address _____

City_____State_____Zip _____

      □   Visa   □   Master Card   □   Am. Express

Credit card number _____Expiration date _____

Order by credit card, personal check or money order. Send to:

Addicus Books
Mail Order Dept.
P.O. Box 45327
Omaha, NE 68145
Or, order TOLL FREE: **800-352-2873**